NONINVASIVE

POSITIVE PRESSURE

VENTILATION:

PRINCIPLES AND APPLICATIONS

Edited by

Nicholas S. Hill, M.D.
Professor of Medicine
Brown University
Director, Critical Care Services
Pulmonary and Critical Care Medicine
Rhode Island Hospital

Providence, Rhode Island, USA

Futura Publishing Company, Inc.
Armonk, NY

Library of Congress Cataloging-in-Publication Data
    Noninvasive positive pressure ventilation: principles and applications / edited by Nicholas S. Hill.
        p. ; cm.
    Includes bibliographical references and index.
    ISBN 0-87993-459-X (alk. paper)
    1. Intermittent positive pressure breathing. 2. Respiratory therapy. I. Hill, Nicholas S., 1949–
    [DNLM: 1. Intermittent Positive-Pressure Ventilation. WF 145 N813 2000]
    RM161 .N66 2000
    615.8′36--dc21

                                                                00-062272

Published by
Futura Publishing Company
135 Bedford Road
Armonk, New York 10504

LC#: 00-062272
ISBN#: 0-87993-459-X

Contributors

Nicolino Ambrosino, M.D. Lung Function and Respiratory Rehabilitation Unit, Salvatore Maugeri Foundation, IRCCS, Medical Center of Gussago (BS), Italy

Mark W. Elliott, M.D., M.R.C.P. St. James's University Hospital, Leeds, United Kingdom

Peter C. Gay, M.D. Division of Pulmonary and Critical Care Medicine, Mayo Clinic, Rochester, Minnesota, USA

Dean Hess, Ph.D., R.R.T. Pulmonary and Critical Care Medicine, Massachusetts General Hospital, Boston, Massachusetts, USA

Nicholas S. Hill, M.D. Pulmonary and Critical Care Medicine, Rhode Island Hospital, Providence, Rhode Island, USA

DeLynn Johnston, B.S., R.R.T. Mallinckrodt, Inc., St. Louis, Missouri, USA

David M. Lang, M.D. John Hopkins University School of Medicine, Division of General Pediatrics and Adolescent Medicine, Baltimore, Maryland, USA

Patrick Leger, M.D. Service de Pneumologie, Centre Medical Eduard Rist, Paris, France

W. Gerald Teague, M.D. Emory School of Medicine, Atlanta, Georgia, USA

Michele Vitacca, M.D. Lung Function and Respiratory Rehabilitation Unit, Salvatore Maugeri Foundation, IRCCS, Medical Center of Gussago (BS), Italy

Foreword

Noninvasive ventilation, particularly nasal positive pressure ventilation, has had a major impact on the care of patients with acute and chronic ventilatory failure in the last two decades. The role of noninvasive positive pressure ventilation (NPPV) in acute exacerbations of chronic obstructive pulmonary disease is now confirmed by evidence-based medicine,[1] and noninvasive positive pressure modes are seen increasingly as valid treatment options in other causes of acute respiratory failure such as pneumonia, cardiogenic pulmonary edema, and respiratory insufficiency following surgery. A recent survey[2] of domiciliary ventilation in the United States showed that nearly 50% of the growth in this area can be attributed to nasal positive pressure ventilation. Here too, the application of noninvasive ventilation is extending to new territories, including use in the 24-hour ventilator-dependent patient and in the pediatric age range. As a result, an increasing range of health care professionals including pulmonologists, respiratory therapists, intensivists, anethesiologists, emergency room staff, pediatricians, neurologists, rehabilitation specialists, and nursing personnel need to be familiar with the indications for nasal positive pressure ventilation, the practicalities of successful implementation, and the limitations. This book provides a superlative state of the art guide to nasal positive pressure ventilation, and is a highly valuable bedside tool for all those involved in the field.

Dr. Nicholas S. Hill, who edited the volume and contributed to many of the chapters, is a pioneer and world-renowned exponent of noninvasive ventilation. He has researched many applications of NPPV with the aim of answering the key questions: does it work, who benefits, and how is the benefit achieved? This book provides the reader with a thorough understanding of the rationale for NPPV, and its advantages and potential drawbacks, compared with other ventilatory approaches.

The important practical issues of equipment selection, matching it to the patient's ventilatory requirements, initiation of therapy, and monitoring are covered lucidly and comprehensively by Drs. Hess, Gay, and Hill. The respective chapters are crucial reading for the novice to noninvasive ventilation and experienced practitioner, alike.

Drs. Ambrosino and Vitacca are well known for their work on the treatment of acute respiratory failure in chronic obstructive pulmonary disease using NPPV, negative pressure ventilation, and conventional invasive techniques. They are well qualified to discuss which acute chronic obstructive pulmonary disease patients are likely to benefit from noninvasive modes, the physiological effects of noninvasive ventilation, and long-term outcome.

Drs. Leger and Hill then examine the use of NPPV in its most long-standing application—chronic respiratory failure due to restrictive ventilatory disorders and central hypoventilation syndromes. Both authors have recently contributed to a Consensus Conference on the use of noninvasive ventilation in chronic respiratory failure,[3] and they provide an authoritative view, not only of current indications, but also of areas where the value of ventilatory support is evolving, such as progressive neuromuscular disease. This last aspect has special resonance as one of the earliest reports of nasal positive pressure ventilation is in patients with Duchenne's muscular dystrophy.[4]

Dr. Elliott has unique experience in the use of long-term NPPV in chronic obstructive pulmonary disease patients. This controversial area is covered even-handedly and with great clarity. The discussion is a must for those who wish to understand the competing arguments as to whether long-term NPPV combined with long-term oxygen therapy is of value in chronic obstructive pulmonary disease and, if so, which patients *might* benefit.

Pediatric applications of nasal positive pressure ventilation have been explored only relatively recently. Drs. Teague and Lang have extensive experience in this area and succinctly discuss pediatric indications, practical problems, and the outcome of NPPV in children.

Of course, NPPV is not a panacea. As with any other ventilatory technique, it will fail in some situations, and in others, practical problems will limit its efficacy. We can all learn from these difficulties, to our patients' benefit. Dr. Hill is uniquely placed to address practical issues, and I anticipate that many experienced and novice noninvasive ventilation practitioners will find this information invaluable.

Finally, there is evidence that, worldwide, the successful uptake of NPPV is being constrained by problems setting up noninvasive ventilation programs, the training of staff, and funding of equipment. Ms. Johnson and Dr. Hill provide an overview of program development, resource utilization, and staffing, which is vital for all those involved in program planning. Although organizational aspects will inevitably differ between countries, outcome assessment is crucial to every program and the reader is guided towards the most constructive ways of assessing a noninvasive ventilation program.

All in all, this volume is an extremely valuable addition to publications on the rapidly growing and dynamic field of NPPV, and should be available in all units caring for adults and children with respiratory insufficiency.

Anita K. Simonds, M.D, F.R.C.P.
Consultant in Respiratory Medicine
Sleep & Ventilation Unit
Royal Brompton & Harefield NHS Trust
London, United Kingdom

References

1. Keenan SP, Kernerman PD, Cook DJ, et al. The effect of noninvasive positive pressure ventilation on mortality in patients admitted with acute respiratory failure: a meta-analaysis. Crit Care Med 1997;25:1685-1692.
2. Adams AB, Shapiro R, Marinii JJ. Changing prevalence of chronically ventilator-assisted individuals in Minnesota: increases, characteristics, and the use of non-invasive ventilation. Respir Care 1998;43:635-636.
3. Consensus Conference. Clinical indications for noninvasive positive pressure ventilation in chronic respiratory failure due to restrictive lung disease, COPD, and nocturnal hypoventilation: a Consensus conference report. Chest 1999;116:521-534.
4. Rideau Y, Gatin G, Bach J, Gines G. Prolongation of life in Duchenne's muscular dystrophy. Acta Neurol 1983;5:118-124.

Introduction

Evolution of Noninvasive Ventilation

Although an understanding of the gas exchange function of respiration awaited the discoveries of respiratory gases during the 1700s, the vital function of respiration has been apparent to humans since antiquity. References to assisted ventilation are found in the Bible,[1] and primitive resuscitation devices have long been available. Techniques that attempted to force gas into the upper airway via bellows were developed centuries ago, as were more creative methods such as the so-called Dutch method that consisted of chest wall compressions combined with tobacco insufflation per rectum to stimulate breathing.[2]

Positive pressure resuscitation devices were outlawed throughout Europe during the 1800s because of the observation that dogs developed fatal pneumothoraces when experimentally resuscitated using these techniques. This led to the development of a variety of manually powered negative pressure devices that were suitable for ventilatory support over a period of hours. By the early 1900s, the polio epidemics created a need for devices capable of providing more sustained ventilatory support, and the wide availability of electricity offered a readily available power source. Inventors busied themselves creating a variety of ingenious devices, commonly referred to as "body" ventilators, that assisted ventilation by exerting force on various regions of the thorax and/or abdomen.

The Age of "Body" Ventilators

Negative pressure ventilators were the most commonly used mechanical ventilators outside of the anesthesia suite during the first half of the 20th century, and they successfully supported many victims of the polio epidemics.[3,4] The most efficient and widely used of the negative pressure ventilators was the tank ventilator, or "iron lung," described by Drinker and Shaw in 1929.[5] The original Drinker ventilator was impractical, weighing in excess of a ton and requiring several minutes for patient removal, a potentially life-threatening hazard in the event of a power failure. Modifications by J.H. Emerson during the early 1930s, which included the capability of manual operation, provided a safe, reliable, and economical alternative to the original Drinker; the Emerson lung became the standard tank-type negative pressure ventilator for the next several decades. A lawsuit brought by Drinker against Emerson for patent violations was later thrown out when Emerson demonstrated that numerous designs for tank ventilators preceded the Drinker.

The iron lung proved to be a very effective device for ventilatory assistance and saved many patients with paralytic poliomyelitis.[6] However, even the formidable Emerson lung had limitations, including bulk and lack of portability (it weighed 300 kg and was 3 m long and 1 m wide). Furthermore, because it entirely encased the patient's body, it interfered with the administration of nursing care and not uncommonly caused claustrophobic reactions in patients. Accordingly, more compact and portable negative pressure ventilators were developed, including the "shell" or cuirass ventilator, which consisted of a rigid breast plate that was strapped over the chest and abdomen. A negative pressure pump generated an intermittent subatmospheric pressure within the shell, assisting lung expansion. Two cuirass ventilators, the Huxley Chest Respirator and Monahan Portable Respirator, were mass produced and widely used for polio patients until the 1960s.

A further modification of negative pressure ventilation was the "jacket" or "wrap" ventilator, first described as the Tunnicliffe breathing jacket during the 1950s.[7] This consisted of an impermeable jacket, poncho, or body suit that was fitted over the thorax and abdomen and suspended from a plastic or metal cage contained within. The rigid cage prevented collapse of the jacket onto the thorax and abdomen so that a negative pressure could be generated within the jacket. Both the shell and jacket were far more portable than the tank ventilator, but were less efficient because they exerted subatmospheric pressure over a smaller surface area of the chest and abdomen.

Although the cuirass and jacket ventilators were more portable than the tank ventilator, they still required negative pressure pumps weighing 20–30 kg. In addition, because they restricted patient position, they often caused musculoskeletal discomfort, rendering patient adaptation difficult. With the cuirass, skin abrasions and elimination of leaks could also be a problem.[8] In addition, all of the negative pressure ventilators could induce obstructive apneas. This was caused by the application of subatmospheric pressure out of phase with the patient's spontaneous inspiration, leading to upper airway collapse and frequent severe oxygen desaturations in many patients.[9]

Other ingenious approaches to body ventilation that were developed during the polio epidemics included the rocking bed[10] and the intermittent abdominal pressure respirator, or "pneumobelt."[11] Both assist diaphragm motion by utilizing the force of gravity on the abdominal contents and are sometimes referred to as "abdominal pressure ventilators."[12] The technique of rocking was first described by Eve in 1932 when it was used to resuscitate a young child with neuromuscular disease.[13] Subsequently, the technique was adopted by the British Navy as a means of resuscitating drowning victims. During the late 1940s, Wright described the rocking bed as a device to aid breathing in polio victims.[14] The device consisted of a mattress placed on a bed frame that rocked through an arc of approximately 40°, with a fulcrum at hip level. When the bed rocked to the head-down position, the abdominal viscera and hence diaphragm slid cephalad, assisting exhalation, and in the foot-down position, the viscera slid caudad, assisting inhalation. The device proved useful for patients who were attempting to wean from the iron lung, and was used, for many decades, for some patients, after a bout of acute poliomyelitis.[15]

The pneumobelt was invented during the 1930s by Sir William Bragg, the Nobel Prize-winning physicist, who fashioned a pneumatic belt from a football bladder for a friend with muscular dystrophy. The current version of the pneumobelt consists of a rubber bladder held firmly against the abdomen within a strapped-on corset. A positive pressure ventilator intermittently inflates the bladder, compressing the abdominal contents, forcing the diaphragm upward and assisting exhalation. When the bladder deflates, gravity returns the abdominal contents and diaphragm to their original positions, assisting inhalation. The device must be used in at least a 30° sitting position, and is thus most suitable for daytime use as an adjunct to other forms of mechanical ventilation. It is ideal for patients who desire to do desk work, because it leaves the arms and face unencumbered. Both the rocking bed and pneumobelt have limitations, working best in patients with diaphragm weakness or paralysis, but poorly in those with an unfavorable body habitus, such as that caused by severe kyphoscoliosis.

The Proliferation of
Invasive Positive Pressure Ventilation

The deficiencies of body ventilators caused clinicians to seek better alternatives. Invasive positive pressure ventilation had been widely used during the first half of the 20th century, but mainly in anesthesia suites. The gradual shift toward invasive positive pressure ventilation as the main means of supporting patients with acute respiratory failure began during the early 1950s. The signal event occurred in Copenhagen during a severe epidemic of poliomyelitis that caused respiratory paralysis in almost 300 victims over a 3-month period.[16] The six negative pressure ventilators initially available were overwhelmed, and the mortality rate approached 80%. Manually powered invasive positive pressure anesthesia devices were assembled to support many of the victims. Medical students, nurses, and lay people were recruited to provide bag ventilation in round-the-clock shifts, sometimes for weeks on end. Mortality rates were reduced to below 30%, and reports of the Copenhagen experience stimulated interest in the development of electrically powered positive pressure ventilators. During the subsequent 15 years, invasive positive pressure ventilation was used more and more for patients with acute respiratory failure as intensive care units were created. Invasive positive pressure ventilation provided direct access to the airway, facilitated nursing care, and was perceived as more effective than negative pressure ventilation. By the late 1960s, noninvasive ventilators were largely supplanted, relegated to use for occasional patients with chronic respiratory failure due to restrictive thoracic disease, at centers still experienced in their use.

The Emergence of Noninvasive Positive Pressure Ventilation

Pioneers like Alvin Barach evaluated noninvasive positive pressure techniques during the first half of the 20th century, reporting successful application in patients with acute pulmonary edema.[17] However, the approach was used much less often than body ventilation. In 1947, intermittent positive pressure breathing (IPPB) was described and, for the next 30 years, it saw widespread use as a respiratory therapy technique in virtually every patient admitted to acute care hospitals with exacerbations of chronic obstructive pulmonary disease (COPD) or asthma. Although it was capable of assisting ventilation, and early studies demonstrated that it prevented the rise in $PaCO_2$ associated with oxygen administration, it never gained acceptance as a means of assisting ventilation. Instead, it was used mainly for the administration of aerosolized bronchodilator medication for periods of only 10-15 minutes 4 times a day, which was too little to provide significant ventilatory assistance. Further, it was administered via mouthpieces that were not amenable to use for longer periods of time. Also, the ventilators used to power the devices were quite primitive and could not adapt easily to the patient's breathing pattern. Accordingly, the ability of IPPB to reduce the work of breathing was quite limited. When a randomized controlled trial demonstrated that IPPB provided no benefit compared to aerosol delivered by a nebulizer alone,[18] its use in acute care hospitals virtually disappeared.

During this time, long-term noninvasive positive pressure ventilation (NPPV) had been used for polio and other neuromuscular patients at certain centers, dating back to the 1960s.[19] Using mouthpieces held in place by lipseals and attached to portable volume-limited ventilators, this technique was successful in supporting severely compromised neuromuscular patients for many years. However, it never gained wide acceptance, partly because of the difficulty patients sometimes encountered in adapting, and partly because of the lack of experience at most centers. During the early 1980s, investigators in France found that NPPV could be successfully applied via a nasal mask to patients with muscular dystrophy.[20] When nasal masks became widely available commercially for the delivery of continuous positive airway pressure (CPAP) to patients with obstructive sleep apnea, reports of the successful administration of nasal ventilation to patients with chronic respiratory failure due to restrictive thoracic disease began to emerge from centers throughout the world.[20-23] Compared to negative pressure ventilation, this technique offered convenient application, a high level of portability, relatively rapid patient adaptation, and the elimination of obstructive apneas. Compared to invasive positive pressure ventilation, NPPV was much easier and less costly to administer.[24] By virtue of these advantages, NPPV rapidly gained wide acceptance as the ventilator modality of first choice for patients with chronic respiratory failure due to restrictive thoracic disease, as long as airway protection was adequate and the need for ventilatory support was not continuous.

By the late 1980s, reports of the successful application of NPPV for acute respiratory failure, either by oronasal or nasal mask, began appearing.[25,26] The increasing acceptance of NPPV for applications in the acute setting was driven by the perceived advantages over invasive ventilation. By avoiding invasion of the upper airways, NPPV offered the potential of reduced trauma to the upper airway and decreased infectious complications of prolonged intubation such as nosocomial pneumonia or sinusitis. In addition, it enhanced patient comfort by virtue of its ability to preserve speech and eating. In the end, it has the potential of reducing patient morbidity and mortality and lowering health care costs by shortening hospital lengths of stay, all while providing improved patient autonomy and comfort.

In summary, the role of NPPV in both acute and chronic settings has been evolving. Advances in technology have led to ventilators specifically designed for the administration of noninvasive ventilation that include many features to improve effectiveness. More comfortable masks have been developed that enhance patient acceptance and success rates. Studies have been published that provide insights into newer and more effective techniques of administration, and which help to define the patient populations that are most apt to benefit.

Current Perspective and Aims of This Volume

One of the most important developments over the past decade in the field of mechanical ventilation has been the increasing role that NPPV has been assuming in the therapy of both acute and chronic forms of respiratory failure. There can be no question that many recipients of NPPV have benefited from the advantages it offers over invasive or other forms of noninvasive mechanical ventilation. It has assumed a central role in the management of patients with chronic respiratory failure due to restrictive thoracic disorders as well as many patients with central hypoventilatory syndromes. Its role as the ventilatory mode of first choice for selected patients with COPD exacerbations has also gained wide acceptance, and although its precise role must be further defined, evidence is accumulating to demonstrate a role in the support of many patients with non-COPD causes of respiratory failure. The role of NPPV in severe stable COPD patients remains to be defined, although it now appears likely that those with severe CO_2 retention and worsening hypoventilation during sleep stand to benefit.

To reap the potential benefits that NPPV offers, clinicians must acquire knowledge, experience, and skill in its proper application. At the present time, NPPV is greatly underutilized in many medical centers throughout the world, to the detriment of patient care and the optimal use of health care resources. On the other hand, overuse is also a risk if NPPV is used with excessive zeal and given to patients with little or no chance of success. The purpose of the present volume is to provide a concise but thorough resource on the current state of knowledge relating to the proper application of NPPV. The volume starts with chapters on equipment and proper techniques for initiation and monitoring. Subsequent chapters discuss the main indications for NPPV in acute and chronic settings, including an examination of the supporting evidence and guidelines for patient selection. Later chapters provide practical advice for dealing with the inevitable problems that arise during management of patients with NPPV and suggestions for organizing and monitoring outcomes of NPPV programs. It is hoped that this volume will serve as a practical guide for busy clinicians as well as a scholarly source of information relating to current and future NPPV applications.

Acknowledgments

I would like to express my indebtedness to the following individuals who made essential contributions to this volume: Jan Hayden, for her expert secretarial assistance, all of the contributors, Steven Korn, Chairman of the Board, and Marcy Kroll, Production Editor, of Futura Publishing Company, Inc., and last, but not least, my wife Sophia, and daughters, Kyra and Alyssa, for indulging me with time at the word processor.

Nicholas S. Hill, M.D.
Providence, Rhode Island

References

1. St. James Bible, Genesis 2:7.
2. Morch ET. History of mechanical ventilation. In Kirby RR, Smith RA, Desautels DA (eds). Mechanical Ventilation. New York, Churchill Livingstone, New York, 1985, pp 1-58.
3. Woollam CHM. The development of apparatus for intermittent negative pressure respiration. Anaesthesia 1976; 31:537-547.
4. Woollam CHM. The development of apparatus for intermittent negative pressure respiration. Anaesthesia 1976; 31:666-685.
5. Drinker P, Shaw LA. An apparatus for the prolonged administration of artificial respiration. I. Design for adults and children. J Clin Invest 1929; 7:229-247.
6. Hodes HL. Treatment of respiratory difficulty in poliomyelitis. In Poliomyelitis: Papers and Discussions Presented at the Third Intenational Poliomyeliytis Conference. Philadelphia, Lippincott, 1955, pp 91-113.
7. Spalding JMK, Opie L. Artificial respiration with the Tunnicliffe breathing-jacket. Lancet 1958; 1: 613-615.
8. Hill NS. Clinical applications of body ventilators. Chest 1986; 90: 897-905.
9. Hill NS, Redline S, Carskadon MA, et al. Sleep-disordered breathing in patients with Duchenne muscular dystrophy using negative pressure ventilators Chest 1992; 102:1656-1662.
10. Plum F, Whedon GD. The rapid-rocking bed: its effect on the ventilation

of poliomyelitis patients with respiratory paralysis. N Engl J Med 1951; 245:235-240.

11. Adamson JP, Lewis L, Stein JD. Application of abdominal pressure for artificial respiration. JAMA 1959; 169:613-617.

12. Hill NS. Use of negative pressure ventilation, rocking beds, and pneumobelts. Respir Care 1994; 39:532-545.

13. Eve FC. Actuation of the inert diaphragm. Lancet 1932; 2:995.

14. Wright J. The Respiraid rocking bed in poliomyelitis. Am J Nurs 1947; 47:454-455.

15. Sternburg L, Sternburg D. View from the Seesaw. New York, Dodd, Mead and Co, 1986.

16. Lassen HCA. The epidemic of poliomyelitis in Copenhagen, 1952. Proc R Soc Med 1954; 47:67-71.

17. Barach AL, Martin J, Eckman M. Positive pressure respiration and its application to the treatment of acute pulmonary edema. Ann Intern Med 1938; 12:754-795.

18. Intermittent Positive Pressure Breathing Trial Group. Intermittent positive pressure breathing therapy of chronic obstructive pulmonary disease. Ann Intern Med 1983, 99:612-620

19. Alba A, Khan A, Lee M. Mouth IPPV for sleep. Rehab Gazette 1984; 24:47-49.

20. Rideau Y, Gatin G, Bach J, Gines G. Prolongation of life in Duchenne's muscular dystrophy. Acta Neurol 1983; 5:118-124.

21. Kerby GR, Mayer LS, Pingleton SK. Nocturnal positive pressure ventilation via nasal mask. Am Rev Respir Dis 1987; 135:738-740.

22. Ellis ER, Bye PT, Bruderer JW, et al. Treatment of respiratory failure during sleep in patients with neuromuscular disease: positive-pressure ventilation through a nose mask. Am Rev Respir Dis 1987; 135:148-152.

23. Bach JR, Alba AS, Bohatiuk G, et al. Mouth intermittent positive pressure ventilation in the management of post-polio respiratory insufficiency. Chest 1987; 91:859-864.

24. Bach JR, Intintola P, Alba AS, Holland I. The ventilator-assisted individual cost analysis of institutionalization versus rehabilitation and in-home management. Chest 1992; 101:26-30.

25. Meduri GU, Conoscenti CC, Menashe P, et al. Noninvasive face mask ventilation in patients with acute respiratory failure. Chest 1989; 95:865-870.

26. Elliott MW, Steven MH, Phillips GD, et al. Non-invasive mechanical ventilation for acute respiratory failure. BMJ 1990; 300:358-360.

Contents

Chapter 1

Equipment Used for Noninvasive Positive Pressure Ventilation

Dean Hess, Ph.D., R.R.T.

Introduction

The primary equipment needs for noninvasive positive pressure ventilation (NPPV) are a positive pressure ventilator and an interface (a mask or similar appliance to direct pressurized gas from the ventilator into the upper airway). Until recently, equipment for noninvasive ventilation was either custom-made to meet the needs of an individual patient, or adapted from equipment designed for other purposes such as administration of continuous positive airway pressure (CPAP) or invasive mechanical ventilation. Equipment that has been designed specifically for noninvasive ventilation is now commercially available from several manufacturers. This chapter will describe the interfaces, ventilators, and other equipment used to provide NPPV.

Interfaces for Noninvasive Ventilation

The choice of patient interface has a major impact on patient comfort and tolerance during noninvasive ventilation.[1-3] The need to select an appropriate and properly fit mask for the patient cannot be overemphasized. A poorly fitting interface will decrease both clinical effectiveness and patient compliance with this therapy. Commonly used interfaces include nasal and full face masks, other nasal interfaces, and mouthpieces.

Masks

Masks to provide noninvasive ventilation can be either nasal masks, or full face (oronasal) masks that cover both the nose and

From *Noninvasive Positive Pressure Ventilation: Principles and Applications,* edited by Nicholas S. Hill. © 2001, Futura Publishing Company, Inc., Armonk, NY.

mouth, and there are advantages and disadvantages of each (Table 1). Desirable features of a mask for noninvasive ventilation are listed in Table 2. Selecting the correct mask size is critical to the success of noninvasive ventilation.[2]

The mask consists of a cushion to maintain a seal with the skin, an enclosing structure usually consisting of clear plastic that has a standard 15-mm or 22-mm connector to the ventilator circuit, and a means of attaching headgear (or straps) to act as a harness (Figure 1). Although the cushion should minimize air leaks during noninvasive ventilation, it is important to recognize that leaks are common and

Table 1
Potential Advantages and
Disadvantages of Nasal Versus Oronasal Masks

Mask	Advantages	Disadvantages
Nasal	Less risk of aspiration	Mouth leak
	Easier secretion clearance	Higher resistance through nasal passages
	Less claustrophobia	Less effective with nasal obstruction
	Easier speech	Nasal irritation and rhinorrhea
	May be able to eat	Mouth dryness
	Easy to fit and secure	Nasal bridge redness and ulceration
	Less dead space	
Oral	Better oral leak control	Increased dead space
	More effective in mouth breathers	Difficult to maintain adequate seal
		Risk of nasal and facial pressure sores
		Claustrophobia
		Increased aspiration risk
		Increased difficulty speaking and eating
		Asphyxiation with ventilator malfunction
		More difficult to fit

Table 2
Desirable Characteristics of a Mask for Noninvasive Ventilation

Low dead space
Transparent
Lightweight
Easy to secure
Adequate seal with low facial pressure
Disposable or easy to clean
Nonirritating to skin (nonallergenic)
Inexpensive

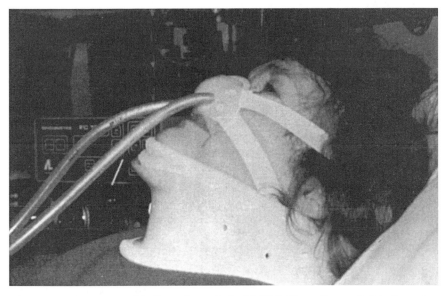

Figure 1. Custom-molded nasal mask for NPPV. (From Leger P. Noninvasive positive pressure ventilation at home. Respir Care 1994;39:501-514.)

may not necessarily compromise the effectiveness of noninvasive ventilation. The cushion should be soft and malleable to the facial anatomy. Several mask cushion styles are used. The traditional cushion available on anesthesia and resuscitation oronasal masks was a hard plastic or air-filled cushion. These are not desirable for noninvasive ventilation because they seal poorly and apply high pressure to the face, which is uncomfortable and increases the likelihood of facial pressure sores.

Newer commercially available masks have open silicone or other soft rubber flanges to achieve an air seal (Figure 1). These masks are designed specifically for noninvasive ventilation, with the cushion pushing harder against the skin as pressure inside the mask increases, tightening the air seal. Some use ultrathin material for the flange so that a good air seal is achieved with minimal strap tension. Recently, several types of masks have become available that use gel-filled flanges (Figure 2) which may improve patient tolerance. Some oronasal masks have soft foam-filled or inflatable air cushions. For the latter, air can be added or removed from the cushion after it is applied to the patient to improve mask fit. With a correctly sized mask, these cushions help to minimize leak and improve comfort during noninvasive ventilation. Complications of masks are discussed in detail in Chapter 10.

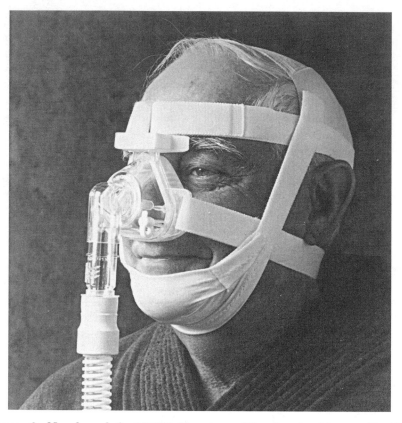

Figure 2. Nasal mask for NPPV. (Courtesy of Respironics, Murrysville, PA.)

Nasal Masks

The nasal mask should fit just above the junction of the nasal bone and cartilage (nasal bridge), and make contact with the skin on the sides of the nasal bridge, the cheek lateral to both nares, and above the upper lip. Use of sizing gauges is recommended to properly fit nasal masks (Figure 1). These sizing gauges are mask-specific and cannot be interchanged between manufacturers or different mask styles of the same manufacturer.

A common mistake is to choose a mask that is too large. This results in leaks, the tendency to excessively tighten the straps to control the leak, decreased effectiveness, and patient discomfort. Use of forehead spacers that come with certain nasal masks is recommended to reduce pressure on the nasal bridge. Many nasal mask styles are now commercially available, including standard nasal CPAP masks, newer minimasks (see below), and masks with gel rather than silicone flanges (Figure 2). In practice, an assortment of various mask styles and sizes should be readily available, so that several masks can be tried to achieve the best fit.

Nasal masks can also be custom-molded for an individual patient (Figure 1),[5-7] but this is generally not necessary because of the variety of sizes and designs of pre-formed masks that are commercially available. Custom masks are molded using silicone putty or heat-sensitive material to form an impression of the patient's face. These may be fabricated from commercially available kits or from materials assembled by practitioners at specialized centers. Theoretically, these should produce a mask that fits the individual anatomy of a patient's face. In practice, however, these are time-consuming and difficult to fabricate, and have virtually no role in NPPV for acute respiratory failure because of the

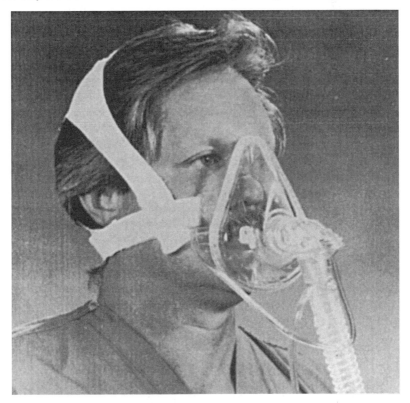

Figure 3. Oronasal mask for NPPV. (From Hill NS. Complications of noninvasive positive pressure ventilation. Respir Care 1997;42:432-442.)

time required for construction. For chronic respiratory failure, custom-molded masks may have a role in the practice of clinicians who have developed the skills required to mold a functional mask for the occasional patient who is unable to tolerate pre-formed masks.

Leaks through the mouth are common when using a nasal mask (see Chapter 10). Typically, these are more problematic during acute respiratory failure than during chronic applications. Mouth leaks should be minimized because their presence has been associated with failure of NPPV[8] and increased nasal resistance.[9] Mouth leaks can be avoided by coaching the patient to keep the mouth closed, use of chin straps, or use of an oronasal mask.

Nasal masks are the most commonly used for chronic applications of NPPV because they are compact in size, they leave the mouth unencumbered for speech, eating, coughing, and oral suctioning, and they minimize claustrophobic reactions (Table 1).

Full Face (Oronasal) Masks

The oronasal mask should fit from just above the junction of the nasal bone and cartilage to the chin just below the lower lip (Figure 3). As with the nasal mask, it is critically important to choose a mask of the correct size to avoid leaks, patient discomfort, and decreased effectiveness. Sizing gauges that are specific to mask type are available to properly fit oronasal masks. Custom-molded oronasal masks can be fabricated (Figure 4) but this is rarely necessary because of the increasing variety of commercial masks available.

Advances in oronasal masks have led to masks specifically designed for noninvasive ventilation, consisting of compact, clear plastic units to minimize dead space and claustrophobic reactions. They also include soft silicone seals to minimize patient discomfort and the development of nasal bridge ulcers. Oronasal masks minimize air leaks through the mouth because they cover both the nose and mouth; however, maintaining a good seal between the chin and silicone seal may be difficult, particularly in edentulous patients. Since acutely dyspneic patients are commonly perceived to be "mouth-breathers," and oronasal masks are thought to minimize air leaks through the mouth, they have gained popularity as the initial mask to use for patients with acute respiratory failure. It should be borne in mind, however, that no published trials have directly compared oronasal and nasal masks in the acute setting, and trials on NPPV for acute respiratory failure have reported similar success rates regardless of the type of mask that is used.

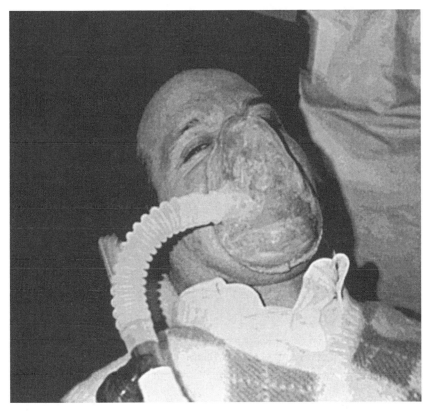

Figure 4. Custom-molded strapless oronasal mask for NPPV. (From Bach JR, Saporito LR. Indications and criteria for decannulation and transition from invasive to noninvasive long-term ventilatory support. Respir Care 1994;39:515-531.)

The greatest concerns related to the use of an oronasal mask are aspiration, should vomiting occur, and asphyxiation (due to rebreathing), in the event of a ventilator malfunction. Commercially available oronasal masks are now available with non-rebreathing valves and quick-release features. Even with this design, close patient monitoring is prudent whenever an oronasal mask is used to provide noninvasive ventilation for acute respiratory failure. Air leaks also commonly occur with oronasal mask ventilation because of the difficulty in sealing over the mandible. Another concern is that the volume of the oronasal mask can contribute to rebreathing and some investigators have reduced this potential dead space by placing a foam insert into the mask.[4] However, this is generally not done in clinical practice, the contribution of the

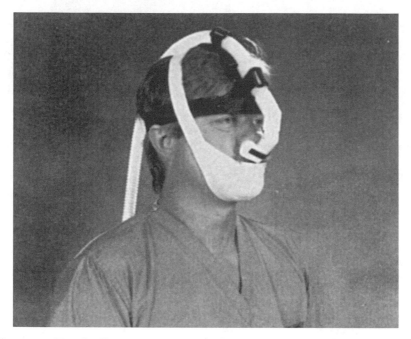

Figure 5. Nasal pillows for NPPV. (From Hill NS. Complications of noninvasive positive pressure ventilation. Respir Care 1997;42:432-442.)

oronasal mask to dead space has not been evaluated in published studies, and its importance is unclear.

Other Nasal Interfaces

Nasal "pillows" or "seals" consist of two small cone-shaped cushions that are inserted directly into the nares for application of pressurized gas (Figure 5). "Minimasks" apply soft silicone seals only to the skin surrounding the openings of the nares on the inferior surface of the nose (Figure 6). Both of these types leave the nasal bridge free, thus either may be used as an alternative to standard nasal masks when patients become intolerant due to excessive pressure or ulceration over the nasal bridge. They may also improve tolerance of NPPV in claustrophobic patients, and permit the use of eyeglasses in patients with impaired eyesight who wish to read or watch television while using NPPV. For these reasons, these interfaces may be advantageous for some patients receiving long-term NPPV. Occasionally, patients may alternate between one of these interfaces and standard nasal masks

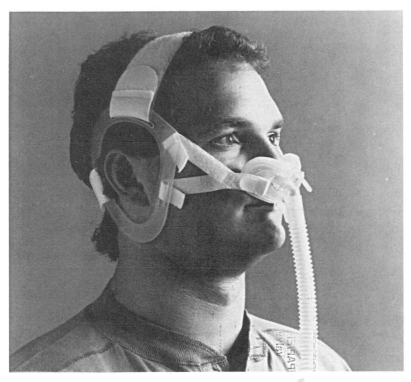

Figure 6. Monarch nasal mask for NPPV. (Courtesy of Respironics, Murrysville, PA.)

to enhance comfort and convenience. The minimask is not recommended for acute applications of noninvasive ventilation, however, because of limited experience and the concern that it is a less stable interface than a standard mask.

Oral Interfaces

Mouthpieces

Although they are almost never used for acute respiratory failure except to facilitate initiation, mouthpieces (Figure 7) and related devices have been used successfully in chronic noninvasive ventilation of patients with neuromuscular diseases.[10-12] These are typically strapless devices that can be held in place using the hands, kept in the mouth using an orthodontic retainer, or attached to a wheelchair via a goose-

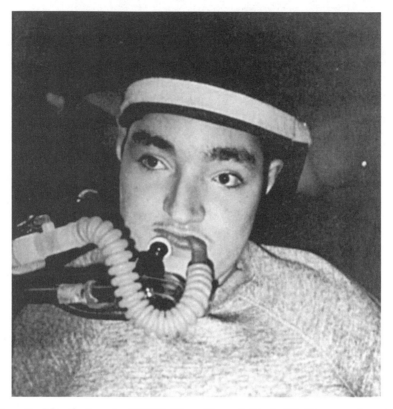

Figure 7. Mouthpiece for NPPV. (From Dean S, Bach JR. The use of noninvasive respiratory muscle aids in the management of patients with progressive neuromuscular diseases. Respir Care Clin North Am 1996;2:223-240.)

neck clamp. They are used mainly at centers with extensive experience in applying them to patients with slowly progressive neuromuscular diseases.[10] They may be a useful alternative for patients with uncontrolled air leaks through the mouth during nasal ventilation, but air leaks through the nose may still occur. Mouthpieces may also cause hypersalivation, and initial adaptation may be difficult. However, once adaptation is successful, mouthpieces provide reliable interfaces that have been used to support patients for many years, even some who have vital capacities that approach zero.[10] Also, because they can easily be expectorated, they do not interfere with speaking or eating. In quadriplegic patients, use of a mouthpiece can interfere with activities that require use of a mouthstick control; over a long period of time, it can also cause orthodontic deformity.

Lipseals

For patients who cannot retain a mouthpiece alone, a lipseal can be added to the mouthpiece (Figure 8). The lipseal is a plastic flange that fits over the mouth and lips and is held in place with straps or headgear, creating an air seal around the mouthpiece. The lipseal is less acceptable than other interfaces for some patients because it interferes with speaking, eating, and secretion clearance. Custom-molded mouthpieces can also be used in which a plastic lipseal is retained by a bite block. These circumvent some of the limitations by maintaining an air seal without the need for straps or headgear, and the patient can quickly expectorate the mouthpiece if the need arises. However, the bite block can stimulate gagging or hypersalivation in some patients.

Headgear

A strap system (or headgear) is needed to maintain correct position of most interfaces and is important for patient comfort. Many varieties

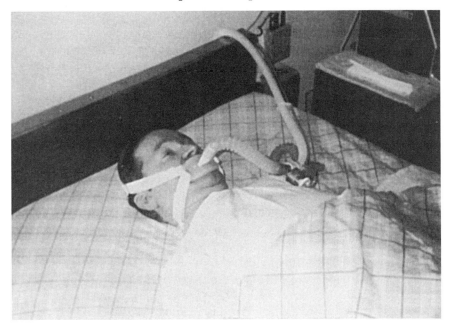

Figure 8. Mouthpiece with lipseal for NPPV. (From Dean S, Bach JR. The use of noninvasive respiratory muscle aids in the management of patients with progressive neuromuscular diseases. Respir Care Clin North Am 1996;2:223-240.)

of headgear are available, but most are designed for a particular interface, so once a mask is chosen, the headgear selection is limited. For short-term use, simple disposable Velcro® straps are most often used, but for long-term applications, more elaborate strap systems attached to caps are often used.

Most interfaces designed specifically for noninvasive ventilation are secured using a combination of cloth or elastic straps, Velcro, and clips. The straps fit through slots or attach to clips at the sides and top of the mask. The number of attachments varies from two to five, depending on mask type. The more numerous the attachments, the more stable the mask, but the more complicated it is to attach. Use of Velcro to secure the mask allows nearly infinite adjustments of the headgear. Once the Velcro is adjusted, detachable clips can be used for rapid removal or replacement. Some oronasal masks use elastic straps with holes that attach to hooks to secure the masks. The hooks can be either on the outer edge of the mask or, more commonly, near the center of the mask. Attachment of the headgear to the outer edge of the mask may better distribute the pressure of the mask and facilitate a seal.

A common mistake is to tighten the headgear excessively in an attempt to eliminate air leaks. To avoid this, it should be possible to pass one or two fingers between the headgear and the face. Fitting the headgear too tightly may even worsen air leak, and always decreases patient comfort and compliance. To minimize air leak, it is advisable to first pull out on the mask and reseat the silicone flange.

Interface Selection

The choice of a particular interface depends on many factors, including practitioner and patient preferences, patient characteristics, and availability. In the acute setting, commercially available disposable nasal or oronasal interfaces are usually chosen, often based on practitioner bias and cost considerations. In the chronic setting, where long-term comfort is more important, selection is based more on patient comfort and mask durability and less on cost, with custom-molded masks and mouthpiece interfaces reserved for patients who fail to tolerate standard masks. Although arguments in favor of one interface over another can be touted and many practitioners have strong biases, few controlled studies comparing interfaces have been published. Thus, interface selection should be based on consideration of the advantages and disadvantages of a particular mask type as well as individual patient factors, such as the tendency to mouth breathe or leak air through the mouth. Selection is largely a trial and error process that aims to optimize patient comfort while delivering effective ventilatory assistance.

Ventilators for Noninvasive Ventilation

Various ventilator types have been used to provide noninvasive ventilation including "critical care" ventilators designed for invasive ventilation in critically ill patients, "home care" ventilators designed for invasive ventilation administered at home, and ventilators designed specifically to provide noninvasive ventilation. Similar rates of success have been reported regardless of the ventilator used.[13] Perhaps more important is that clinicians understand the functions and limitations of the particular ventilator during use for noninvasive ventilation.

Terminology

Ventilators designed specifically to provide noninvasive ventilation are usually pressure-limited devices, many of which deliver so-called "bilevel" ventilation similar to pressure support ventilation (Figure 9). These ventilators deliver a higher inspiratory pressure when triggered by the patient, which has been referred to as IPAP (inspiratory positive airway pressure). They cycle into expiration, usually after sensing a reduction in inspiratory flow (as with pressure support) or reaching an inspiratory time limit, and deliver a lower expiratory pressure that is referred to as EPAP (expiratory positive airway pressure). IPAP is the absolute inspiratory pressure and is the sum of the expiratory pressure and the increase during inspiration. This terminology differs from that of most critical care ventilators, where the inspiratory pressure, often referred to as pressure support, is the difference between absolute inspiratory and expiratory pressures. In addition, with these ventilators, EPAP is synonymous with positive end-expiratory pressure (PEEP).

Tidal breaths during noninvasive positive pressure breathing can be described by the variables that trigger the breath (the *trigger* variable), govern gas flow (the *limit* or *target* variable), and terminate the breath (the *cycle* variable).[1] Common breath types during noninvasive ventilation are:

- pressure support: patient-triggered, pressure-limited, flow-cycled

- pressure assist: patient-triggered, pressure-limited, time-cycled

- pressure control: machine-triggered, pressure-limited, time-cycled

- volume assist: patient-triggered, flow-limited, volume-cycled

- volume control: machine-triggered, flow-limited, volume-cycled

Ventilators that deliver *bilevel positive airway pressure* combine pressure-limited breaths during inspiration with PEEP. These ventilators may be capable of delivering a variety of modes including CPAP, pressure support (spontaneous or S mode), pressure control (timed or T mode), pressure assist, and pressure support with a backup rate (spontaneous/timed or S/T mode).

Critical Care Ventilators

Critical care ventilators have traditionally been used only for invasive ventilatory support in critically ill patients, but can be used for noninvasive ventilation by attaching the circuit to a mask rather than an endotracheal tube. This approach has the advantages of precise control of fraction of inspired oxygen (FiO_2), a choice of inspiratory flow patterns and pressure- or volume-limited modes, and separation of inspiratory and expiratory ventilator tubing to minimize rebreathing. Critical care ventilators have extensive monitoring and alarm capabilities which are desirable during invasive ventilation, but can be distracting and annoying (for patients and clinicians alike) during noninvasive ventilation. Although critical care ventilators are more expensive than portable ventilators, one might argue that this is not important unless the hospital inventory of critical care ventilators can be reduced as the result of noninvasive ventilation. Perhaps the greatest disadvantage of critical care ventilators is their difficulty in dealing with air leaks that invariably occur during noninvasive ventilation.

Pressure support can be problematic when noninvasive ventilation is provided with a critical care ventilator. Critical care ventilators cycle to the expiratory phase during pressure support when the flow decreases to a ventilator preset level (e.g., 5 L/min or 25% of peak inspiratory flow). If the leak is greater than the flow at which the ventilator cycles, then the patient's exhalation will not be sensed, inspiration will be prolonged, and patient-ventilator dyssynchrony will occur.[14] To

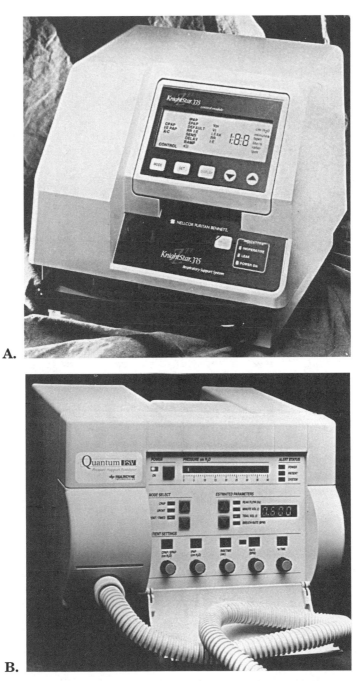

Figure 9. Portable "bilevel" ventilators for NPPV. **A.** Mallinckrodt KnightStar 335. (Courtesy of Mallinckrodt, Inc., St. Louis, MO.) **B.** Respironics Quantum PSV. (Courtesy of Respironics, Inc., Murrysville, PA.) *(Continued.)*

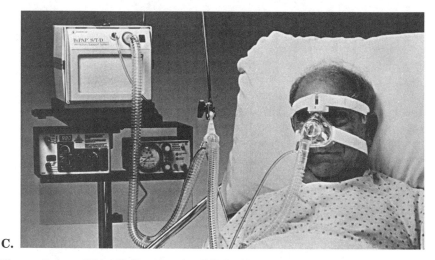

C.

Figure 9 (cont'd.). C. Respironics S/T-D. (Courtesy of Respironics, Murrysville, PA.)

overcome this problem, pressure assist with a short inspiratory time (1–1.5 sec) can be used rather than pressure support. Even without a leak, patients with chronic obstructive pulmonary disease (COPD) using pressure support with a critical care ventilator may have a prolonged ventilator inspiratory time that leads to patient-ventilator asynchrony[15] because of a breathing pattern that is characterized by high inspiratory flow rates for a brief duration. As is the case for those with leaks, these patients may also benefit from pressure assist with a short inspiratory time instead of pressure support.

Portable Volume-Limited Ventilators

Portable volume-limited home care ventilators have long been used to provide noninvasive ventilation, particularly for patients with neuromuscular diseases. These ventilators tend to work well when there is little patient-ventilator interaction, such as during sleep in patients with neuromuscular disease who often allow the ventilator to control their breathing. Generally, the trigger on these ventilators is relatively insensitive and inspiratory flow is fixed. This limits their use for noninvasive ventilation during acute respiratory failure, although success has been reported for this application as well. Like critical care ventilators, these ventilators generally do not tolerate large leaks, although to some extent, compensation for leaks can be made by increasing the delivered tidal volume. These ventilators generally offer only assist/ control or synchronized intermittent mandatory ventilation and monitor only inspiratory pressure, but have a substantial number of alarms. Partly because they include an internal battery, they are fairly heavy, weighing 15–20 kg, but the battery is desirable for home use. They also have separate inspiratory and expiratory tubing, so carbon dioxide (CO_2) rebreathing is not a problem.

Portable Pressure-Limited Ventilators

Often referred to as bilevel ventilators, these are blower-based systems that evolved from CPAP devices (Figure 9). The addition of a valve system permitted cycling from lower expiratory to higher inspiratory pressures and allowed these devices to function as pressure-limited ventilators. Their major advantages are that they are lightweight (3–10 kg), economical, and capable of compensating for air leaks. In fact, they function correctly only in the presence of an air leak. Although they can be used to provide controlled ventilation in the absence of patient effort, they are usually used to provide pressure assist or pressure support ventilation. These ventilators typically provide no higher than modest inspiratory (30 cm H_2O) and expiratory (20 cm H_2O) pressures, and they have relatively limited alarm and monitoring capabilities. Recommendations for the performance of these devices have been published in the form of a consensus statement.[1] Laboratory and clinical evaluations of these devices have been published.[16-20] These studies demonstrate that triggering and flow-generating capabilities of these ventilators compare favorably with those of critical care ventilators.

Two important issues relevant to how well these ventilators function are triggering into the inspiratory phase and cycling into the expiratory phase. Some bilevel ventilators automatically adjust the inspiratory trigger and expiratory cycle by tracking the patient's inspiratory and expiratory flows. Others allow the clinician to adjust the trigger and/or cycle sensitivity. The ability to adjust the trigger sensitivity allows the clinician to balance the ability of the patient to initiate the inspiratory phase against the tendency of the ventilator to auto-cycle. In adjusting the cycle sensitivity, the practitioner aims for a balance between premature termination of the inspiratory phase and delayed cycling requiring that the patient activate expiratory muscles in order to terminate the inspiratory phase.

As is the case with the pressure support mode delivered using critical care ventilators, prolonged exhalation and difficulty with expiratory cycling can also be problematic, particularly in patients with COPD.[15] With high airway resistance and lung compliance (e.g., COPD), flow decelerates slowly with pressure ventilation, producing a prolonged inspiratory phase when the flow at which inspiration terminates is low. When adjustments are possible, both inspiratory trigger and expiratory cycle should be set to optimize patient-ventilator synchrony.

Rebreathing

Another issue that has generated considerable attention with bilevel ventilators is the potential for CO_2 rebreathing.[21-23] Most bilevel ventilators use a single tube without a true exhalation valve (Figure 10). Expired gas passes through a fixed opening that is incorporated into the interface, ventilator tubing, or in a device placed between the ventilator tubing and interface. Particularly with low flow from the ventilator, as may occur with low PEEP levels, there may be inadequate flushing of CO_2 through the opening, leading to rebreathing. This is of particular concern for patients with hypercapnic respiratory failure and has been described mainly with the BiPAP™ (Respironics, Inc., Murrysville, PA) device. The problem can be ameliorated by use of higher PEEP levels so that more CO_2 is flushed from the system, or by use of an exhalation valve that prevents rebreathing. If a non-rebreathing valve is used, it should not increase expiratory resistance or interfere with triggering or cycling of the ventilator.

Alarms and Monitoring

The appropriate role of alarms and monitoring for bilevel devices is controversial. Many patients receiving long-term noninvasive ventilation can sustain adequate spontaneous breathing for hours at a time without ventilatory assistance, but for those capable of only brief ventilator-free periods, disconnect and power-loss alarms are recommended.[1] Also, monitoring of airway pressure and tidal volume are unnecessary for long-term applications, but are desirable for patients with acute respiratory failure. On the other hand, sophisticated monitoring of ventilator parameters is probably unnecessary, because NPPV is generally used for partial rather than complete ventilatory support, and because the ubiquity of leaks makes accurate monitoring of delivered volumes quite difficult. More important is the level of patient monitoring that is dictated by the acuity of illness.

Newer Ventilators and
Modes for Noninvasive Ventilation

Technological advances in mechanical ventilators are rendering some of the earlier concerns about ventilator selection moot. Newer ventilators offer modifications that attempt to improve patient-ventilator synchrony. Although earlier versions of the BiPAP device would deliver inspiratory times up to 3 sec in the presence of leak, leading to inversion of the inspiratory to expiratory (I:E) ratio and a reduction in assisted tidal volumes,[24] more recent versions incorporate mechanisms designed to detect leak and cycle at more appropriate times. Other ventilators permit adjustment of triggering and cycling sensitivities to deal with this problem (KnightStar 335, Mallinckrodt, Inc., St. Louis, MO) and still others permit the operator to set a maximal inspiratory duration (VPAP ST-A, Resmed, San Diego, CA).

Another group of recently introduced ventilators permits application of features of critical care ventilators not only in the critical care setting, but also in the nonacute setting or home (T Bird Legacy, Thermo Respiratory Group, Palm Springs, CA; LTV 1000, Pulmonetics, Inc., Colton, CA; Achieva, Mallinkrodt, Inc.; and Smartvent 201, Versa Med, Inc., Hackensack, NJ) Most of these ventilators use a high-speed turbine to generate air flow (Achieva is piston-powered) and microprocessor technology to offer a wide variety of modes. These include pressure- and volume-targeted modes such as assist/control, synchronized intermittent mandatory ventilation, pressure support, and CPAP. They also offer adjustable flow or pressure-regulated triggers and O_2 blenders for accurate delivery of high FiO_2. They offer sophisticated alarm and monitoring capabilities and one (Smartvent 201) has a screen for graphic displays. Most are compact and lightweight and can operate with internal or external batteries. The LTV 1000 is notable in this regard in that, by virtue of miniaturization technology, it is contained in a device no larger than a laptop computer and weighs only 12.6 lbs including its internal battery. Although these ventilators offer exciting possibilities, they add to the expense of long-term ventilation and they have not been evaluated in controlled clinical studies for either invasive or noninvasive applications. They also raise the concern that they offer more technological capabilities than are needed for most noninvasive applications, particularly in the home.

A recently developed ventilator mode offers the potential for improved delivery of noninvasive ventilation, at least for certain applications. Proportional assist ventilation (PAV) differs from traditional modes of ventilation in that it targets patient inspiratory flow (as an index of effort) rather than pressure or volume.[25] It does so by providing a signal from an in-line flow meter to the ventilator, giving instantaneous feedback on patient breathing demand. If the patient generates more inspiratory flow, the ventilator responds by providing more pressure and flow to assist ventilation. It is possible to adjust the proportion of flow or pressure provided to the patient, so that ventilatory assistance can be partial or complete. By responding to patient effort in this manner, PAV is able to respond instantaneously to changes in patient breathing demand or pattern, and offers the potential of improved synchrony and comfort compared with traditional modes. These properties are particularly attractive for administration of noninvasive ventilation in the acute setting, when the ability to rapidly and comfortably relieve respiratory distress may be important. A recent preliminary trial compared noninvasive PAV to pressure support for patients with acute respiratory insufficiency. In this trial, patients treated with PAV had a greater initial reduction of respiratory rate, refused therapy less often, and had higher mask comfort ratings than those treated with pressure support, which was consistent with the idea that PAV enhances patient comfort.[26] This mode is available on the Vision™ ventilator (Respironics, Inc.) outside of the United States, but it has not yet been approved by the Food and Drug Administration.

Ventilator Circuits

For critical care and portable volume ventilators, the circuit (or tubing) remains the same regardless of whether invasive or noninvasive ventilation is being delivered. The difference is that the circuit is attached to a noninvasive interface (e.g., mask or mouthpiece) rather than an invasive airway (e.g., endotracheal or tracheostomy tube). The portable bilevel pressure-limited ventilators, on the other hand, use a single hose that has a low-resistance smooth-bore inner surface. Two features of this circuit are particularly important. First, the resistance through the circuit must be low. Otherwise, the controllers within the ventilator will not be able to precisely control pressure and flow at the patient interface. Second, these ventilators are designed to function with a fixed leak that is incorporated into the circuit or interface and also functions as the exhalation port for the patient. Because this leak is crucial for the proper triggering and cycling of a particular ventilator as well as control of rebreathing, circuits and interfaces are not inter-changeable among manufacturers.

Miscellaneous Equipment

Oxygen Administration

For critical care ventilators, supplemental oxygen during NPPV can be administered accurately via the oxygen blender just as for invasive ventilation. For portable ventilators, oxygen administration is not so straightforward. Portable volume ventilators typically provide supplemental oxygen by attachment of an oxygen accumulator to the gas entry port or by the titration of oxygen into the inspiratory limb between the ventilator and the humidifier. Oxygen enters the accumulator and is drawn into the ventilator inlet with room air to achieve the desired FiO_2. Supplemental oxygen can also be increased by the use of an oxygen delivery elbow between the ventilator and the humidifier. A more stable FiO_2 is possible with the accumulator than with the oxygen delivery elbow. Also, the bias flow with the oxygen elbow increases the effort necessary to trigger the ventilator and increases the delivered tidal volume.

For bilevel ventilators, supplemental O_2 is provided via a nipple in the mask or a T-tube placed in the circuit at the ventilator outlet (Figure 10). Liter flow is then adjusted to maintain a desired O_2 saturation or tension. Administration of a precise FiO_2 is nearly impossible with the portable pressure-limited ventilators because FiO_2 varies as the ventilatory pattern changes. Due to the high inspiratory airflows from these ventilators, it is difficult to achieve an FiO_2 greater than 0.50. Other ventilators are usually preferred in patients with severe oxygenation defects, although some of the newer bilevel ventilators (Vision^{TM}, Respironics) have oxygen blenders.

Humidification

When critical care ventilators are used, upper airway dryness may be more problematic compared with portable pressure ventilators. This is because critical care ventilators deliver positive pressure from a dry gas source, whereas portable pressure ventilators use ambient air. Gas humidification is not obligatory with noninvasive ventilation because the upper airway is not bypassed, as is the case with invasive ventila-

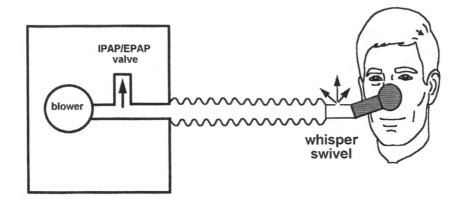

Figure 10. Schematic illustration of a noninvasive positive pressure ventilator. Airway pressure is generated with a blower and controlled by valves within the ventilator. The whisper swivel provides a fixed leak and an exhalation port (incorporated into the mask in some designs). Oxygen can be titrated into the hose at the outlet of the ventilator or into the mask.

tion. However, some patients complain of nasal and/or oral drying during noninvasive ventilation, particularly those who use NPPV chronically in northern climates during the winter months.[2] Oral dryness during nasal ventilation is also often due to mouth leaks, and efforts to minimize the leak (e.g., chin straps, oronasal masks) often correct this problem. Nasal drying may respond to topical saline drops or emollient sprays. Nasal congestion may respond to topical steroids or decongestants.

For patients who remain uncomfortable despite these measures, the inspired gas is humidified. However, heated humidifiers are rarely needed. When a humidifier is added to the circuit of a noninvasive ventilator, it is important to assure that it does not affect the ability of the patient to trigger or cycle the ventilator. This is of particular concern with heat and moisture exchangers, which should not be used with noninvasive ventilation. Patients using portable pressure-limited ventilators should use only pass-over humidifiers recommended by the manufacturer, because pass-through type humidifiers may interfere with triggering and reduce delivered pressure.

Secretion Clearance

Secretion clearance can be critically important for patients requiring noninvasive ventilatory support, particularly those with neuromuscular disease and weakened cough muscles. NPPV may improve secretion clearance in some patients, much like intermittent positive pressure breathing (IPPB). For patients who are troubled by secretion retention, particularly those with neuromuscular disease, assisted cough techniques should be used. Postural drainage and manually assisted (or quad) coughing techniques should be initiated, and other techniques including the forced exhalation technique and autogenic drainage should be considered.[27]

Mechanical devices to improve secretion clearance include the flutter valve, the intrapulmonary percussive ventilator, high-frequency chest wall compression, and the In-Exsufflator (JH Emerson, Cambridge, MA) (Figure 11).[28] This device delivers a high positive inspiratory pressure (e.g., 30–40 cm H_2O) for 1–2 sec via a face mask, followed immediately by a negative pressure (e.g. –30–40 cm H_2O). The intent is to simulate a cough. The level and duration of positive and negative pressures are set by the clinician. The therapy is typically administered as 4–6 positive-negative cycles, which are followed by a period of quiet

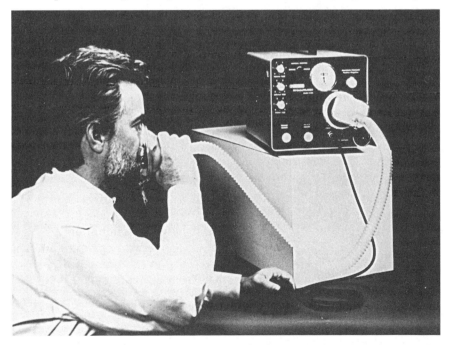

Figure 11. In-Exsufflator. (Courtesy of JH Emerson, Cambridge, MA.) An oronasal mask provides the interface between the patient and the device. The In-Exsufflator provides a high positive pressure followed immediately by a low negative pressure to simulate a cough.

breathing and secretion removal from the mouth and upper airway. The therapy may be repeated as necessary, as dictated by secretion production. Use of this therapy has been associated with a reduced need for hospitalization in neuromuscular patients, but it should be used with caution in patients with COPD, because the negative pressure during expiration may promote airway closure.

Aerosol Medication Delivery

A practical issue during NPPV is how to deliver inhaled medications. Usually the patient can be removed from the ventilator for nebulizer or inhaler therapy and replaced before significant clinical deterioration occurs. However, some patients deteriorate even during brief interruptions. When critical care ventilators are used, the nebulizer control on the ventilator can be used. With bilevel ventilators, a nebulizer can be placed between the mask and the hose from the ventilator.[29] There may be considerable drug loss on the face and in the nose, but this may not affect the bronchodilator response.[30] Unfortunately, there are few data to guide practice in this area, and there is currently no ideal solution to this practical problem.

Summary and Conclusions

Optimal administration of noninvasive ventilation requires knowledge of and experience with the proper application of the equipment required. Also, because advances are continually being made, the knowledge base must be frequently updated. Nasal and oronasal masks are the most commonly used for noninvasive ventilation—nasal for chronic applications, and oronasal more frequently for acute applications. Both masks have advantages and disadvantages, but neither has been shown to be superior to the other in controlled trials. Proper fitting and application is key to the success of noninvasive ventilation. Numerous different types of ventilators are also available for administration of noninvasive ventilation. Critical care or bilevel ventilators have been used for most of the reports in the literature, but neither type has demonstrated superiority over the other in controlled trials. The choice of the particular ventilator is probably not as important as obtaining a proper mask fit and making appropriate adjustments in ventilator settings. Further, newer bilevel ventilators have improved monitoring and alarm capabilities, and include an oxygen blender.

During the past 15 years, the equipment available for noninvasive ventilation has advanced markedly. We can expect that these technological advances will continue, and thus clinicians must keep abreast of the changes to offer optimal noninvasive systems to their patients.

References

1. Bach JR, Brougher P, Hess DR, et al. Consensus statement: noninvasive positive pressure ventilation. Respir Care 1997;42:365-369.
2. Hill NS. Complications of noninvasive positive pressure ventilation. Respir Care 1997;42:432-442.
3. Turner RE. Patient-interface issues in noninvasive positive pressure ventilation. Respir Care 1997;42:389-393.
4. Brochard L, Mancebo J, Wysocki M, et al. Noninvasive ventilation for acute exacerbations of chronic obstructive pulmonary disease. N Engl J Med 1995;333:817-822.
5. Leger P. Noninvasive positive pressure ventilation at home. Respir Care 1994;39:501-514.
6. Bach JR, Saporito LR. Indications and criteria for decannulation and transition from invasive to noninvasive long-term ventilatory support. Respir Care 1994;39:515-531.
7. McDermott I, Bach JR, Parker C, et al. Custom-fabricated interfaces for intermittent positive pressure ventilation via nasal mask for patients with neuromuscular weakness or restrictive lung or chest wall disease. Respir Care 1989;34:73-79.
8. Soo Hoo GW, Santiago S, Williams AJ. Nasal mechanical ventilation for hypercapnic respiratory failure in chronic obstructive pulmonary disease: determinants of success and failure. Crit Care Med 1994;22:1253-1261.
9. Richards GN, Cistulli PA, Ungar RG, et al. Mouth leak with nasal continuous positive airway pressure increases nasal airway resistance. Am J Respir Crit Care Med 1996;154:182-186.
10. Bach JR, Alba AS, Saporito LR. Intermittent positive pressure ventilation via the mouth as an alternative to tracheostomy for 257 ventilator users. Chest 1993;103:174-182.
11. Bach JR. Update and perspectives on noninvasive respiratory muscle aids. Part 1: The inspiratory aids. Chest 1994;105:1230-1240.
12. Bach JR. The prevention of ventilatory failure due to inadequate pump function. Respir Care 1997;42:403-413.
13. Hess D. Noninvasive positive pressure ventilation: predictors of success and failure for adult acute care applications. Respir Care 1997;42:424-431.
14. Black JW, Grover BS. A hazard of pressure support ventilation. Chest 1988;93:333-335.
15. Jubran A, van de Graaff WB, Tobin MJ. Variability of patient-ventilator interaction with pressure support ventilation in patients with chronic obstructive pulmonary disease. Am J Respir Crit Care Med 1995;152:129-136.
16. Kacmarek RM. Performance characteristics of portable ventilators used for noninvasive positive pressure ventilation. Respir Care 1997;42:380-388.

17. Strumpf DA, Carlisle CC, Millman RP, et al. An evaluation of the Respironics BiPAP Bilevel CPAP device for delivery of assisted ventilation. Respir Care 1990; 35:415-422.
18. Hill NS, Mehta S, Carlisle CC, et al. Evaluation of the Puritan-Bennett 335 portable pressure support ventilator: comparison with the Respironics BiPAP S/T. Respir Care 1996;41:885-894.
19. Bunburaphong T, Imanaka H, Nishimura M, et al. Performance characteristics of bilevel pressure ventilators: a lung model study. Chest 1997;111:1050-1160.
20. Drinkwine J, Kacmarek RM. Noninvasive positive pressure ventilation: equipment and techniques. Respir Care Clin North Am 1996;2:183-194.
21. Lofaso F, Brochard L, Hang T, et al. Home versus intensive care pressure support devices: experimental and clinical comparison. Am J Respir Crit Care Med 1996;153:1591-1599.
22. Lofaso F, Brochard L, Touchard D, et al. Evaluation of carbon dioxide rebreathing during pressure support ventilation with airway management system (BiPAP) devices. Chest 1995;108:772-778.
23. Ferguson GT, Gilmartin M. CO_2 rebreathing during BiPAP ventilatory assistance. Am J Respir Crit Care Med 1995;151:1126-1135.
24. Meyer TJ, Pressman MR, Benditt J, et al. Air leaking through the mouth during nocturnal nasal ventilation: effect on sleep quality. Sleep 1997;20:561-569.
25. Younes M, Puddy A, Roberts D, et al. Proportional assist ventilation: results of an initial clinical trial. Am Rev Respir Dis 1992;145:121-129.
26. Gay P, Heil D, Hollets S, et al. A randomized, prospective trial of noninvasive proportional assist ventilation (PAV) to treat acute respiratory insufficiency (ARI). Am J Respir Crit Care Med 1999;159:A14.
27. Hardy KA, Anderson BD. Noninvasive clearance of airway secretions. Respir Care Clin North Am 1996;2:323-345.
28. Bach JR. Update and perspective on noninvasive respiratory muscle aids. Part 2: The expiratory aids. Chest 1994;105:1538-1544.
29. Pollack CV, Fleisch KB, Dowsey K. Treatment of acute bronchospasm with beta-adrenergic agonist aerosols delivered by a nasal bilevel positive airway pressure circuit. Ann Emerg Med 1995;26:552-557.
30. Parkes SN, Bersten AD. Aerosol kinetics and bronchodilator efficacy during continuous positive airway pressure delivered by face mask. Thorax 1997;52:171-175.

Chapter 2

Initiation of Noninvasive Positive Pressure Ventilation

Nicholas S. Hill, M.D., Dean Hess, Ph.D., R.R.T.

Introduction

The initiation of noninvasive positive pressure ventilation (NPPV) requires knowledge and skills regarding the technical aspects of mechanical ventilation, as well as patience and the ability to coach patients to adapt to the mask and ventilator. Successful initiation requires that a series of clinical judgments be made based on knowledge and experience as well as close observation of the patient's response. The first judgment is selection of appropriate patients, based on guidelines that will be discussed in more detail in later chapters. Next, a location and personnel for initiation must be identified and an interface and ventilator selected. After mask fitting, appropriate ventilator settings must be chosen, based on the main goals of noninvasive ventilation. This chapter will discuss these important steps in successful clinical application of NPPV, and also review contrasting approaches for the acute and chronic settings.

Goals of Noninvasive Ventilation

Before initiating NPPV, the clinician should formulate a list of individualized patient goals. Ultimately, for most patients, ventilatory assistance is initiated to improve gas exchange abnormalities and to ameliorate associated symptoms (Table 1). These goals should be achieved while optimizing patient safety and minimizing complications. In the acute setting, avoidance of intubation and its attendant complications is often a top priority. Alleviation of respiratory distress and optimization of patient comfort are also high priorities, because patient

From *Noninvasive Positive Pressure Ventilation: Principles and Applications,* edited by Nicholas S. Hill. © 2001, Futura Publishing Company, Inc., Armonk, NY.

Table 1
Goals of Noninvasive Ventilation

Acute Setting
  Alleviate respiratory distress
  Improve gas exchange abnormalities
  Achieve good patient-ventilator synchrony
  Optimize patient comfort
  Reduce work of breathing
  Avert intubation
  Minimize risk
  Avoid complications
Chronic Setting
  Stabilize gas exchange
  Alleviate fatigue/somnolence
  Improve sleep quality
  Improve quality of life
  Avoid complications
  Avoid hospitalization
  Prolong survival

---

cooperation is necessary, the ability to use sedatives or analgesics is limited, and an uncomfortable patient is likely to reject the therapy. Often, the best indicators of success are reduced work of breathing as indicated by a prompt drop in respiratory rate and good synchrony between the patient and ventilator.

With long-term NPPV and depending on the patient, there may be other secondary goals of noninvasive ventilation, i.e., improvement of sleep quality or resting of respiratory muscles. Avoidance of hospitalization and prolongation of survival, as well as improvement in quality of life are also frequent goals. Quality of life considerations may include ease of use and portability of the equipment so that travel is possible. These goals should be borne in mind when making selections of interfaces, ventilators, and ventilator settings.

Selection of Appropriate Patients

Selection of appropriate patients for NPPV is key to successful implementation. Selection guidelines for specific causes of respiratory failure are discussed in more detail in later chapters, but the process will be discussed in general terms here. Key features of appropriate patients are listed in Table 2.

Table 2
Key Features of Appropriate Patients for NPPV

Features	Acute Setting	Chronic Setting
Symptoms	Dyspnea	Morning headache, hypersomnolence, fatigue
Gas exchange	Acute or acute on chronic hypercapnia and/or moderate to severe hypoxemia	Chronic hypercapnia or nocturnal hypoventilation
Cooperation	Not agitated	Motivated
Able to protect airway	No severe cough or swallowing impairment	Judgment based on patient desires regarding intubation
No excessive secretions	No need for frequent suctioning	Able to expectorate with or without assistance
Able to fit mask	No facial trauma or upper airway surgery	No facial deformities that preclude mask fitting

First, appropriate candidates for NPPV have symptoms attributable to their respiratory impairment. Because noninvasive ventilation entails some discomfort and requires effort on the part of the patient for successful adaptation, patients who are motivated by the desire for symptom relief fare best.[1] Asymptomatic patients, even those with gas exchange impairment, rarely have sufficient motivation to use NPPV. It should be borne in mind, however, that some patients with severe gas exchange disturbances initially deny symptoms but still have substantial symptomatic improvement after successful initiation of NPPV. The desire to avoid airway invasion is also a strong motivator and, in the acute setting, this should be verbally reinforced frequently.

In general, patients who are successfully managed with NPPV are cooperative and capable of understanding the purpose of the therapy. In the acute setting, however, lethargic or even stuporous patients can be managed successfully, as long as they do not become excessively agitated. Because NPPV leaves control of the upper airway to the patient, intact swallowing and cough mechanisms are also desirable. On the other hand, some impairment of these functions is permissible, as long as the impairment is not severe. Patients with bulbar involvement due to amyotrophic lateral sclerosis may respond well to NPPV and survive longer than similar patients who are intolerant of noninvasive ventilation.[2] The combination of severe cough and swallowing impairment is usually lethal, however, and patients with these deficits should undergo invasive ventilation if they desire maximum prolongation of survival.

Along these lines, a manageable amount of airway secretions is desirable, although it is difficult to specify the amount. In general, the greater the impairment of cough or swallowing, the smaller the quantity of secretions needed to cause problems. Patients who repeatedly have bouts of hypoxemia or ventilatory failure because of retained secretions despite application of cough assist techniques (see Chapter 1 for details) should be ventilated invasively.

Patients who have facial trauma or anatomic abnormalities that interfere with mask fitting, or who have had upper airway surgery, are poor candidates for NPPV. In general though, with the variety of interfaces available, the vast majority of patients can be successfully fitted with a mask, and attention to the characteristics listed in Table 2 can help to optimize success rates.

Location for Initiation of Noninvasive Ventilation

Success rates and the safety of initiating NPPV depend partly on the selection of an appropriate location. This choice depends on the acuity of the patient's illness as well as the resources available to the clinician. In the absence of studies establishing the superiority of one location over another, a number of options must be considered, and clinical judgment must be used in deciding between them.

Acute Applications

Patients with respiratory distress who present to acute care hospitals are usually started on NPPV in an emergency department and then transferred to another ward. For patients who develop respiratory failure after admission, NPPV can be initiated in almost any setting, but they must then be transferred to an appropriate location. The main determinant of the appropriate site should be the clinician's assessment of the patient's risk for deterioration in the event that unplanned discontinuation occurs. If the patient is likely to deteriorate within minutes after removal of the mask, a closely monitored setting such as an intensive care or step-down unit should be used. However, if the patient breathes adequately without ventilatory assistance for at least 20–30 minutes, a regular medical or surgical ward may be appropriate. A study by Plant et al.[3] has shown that, for selected patients with moderate exacerbations (pH > 7.30), initiation on a general medical ward may be successful when beds in more intensively monitored settings are unavailable.

Chronic Applications

There are many possible choices for the location of initiation of long-term noninvasive ventilation, ranging from the hospital to the home. The choice should be based on the clinician's assessment of the patient's severity of illness and rapidity of progression as well as the patient's desires. Even for patients who are otherwise medically stable, however, a brief hospitalization is sometimes used to initiate noninvasive ventilation.[4] This permits closer observation and monitoring over a period of days, so that patient motivation can be reinforced and mask and ventilator adjustments can be made promptly and frequently. However, hospitalization is expensive, has not been documented to increase patient compliance rates compared with outpatient initiation, and may be impractical because of constraints on hospital bed usage in some countries such as the United States.

Alternatively, noninvasive ventilation may be initiated in a sleep laboratory. This can be done either during a daytime nap study or as part of a "split" nocturnal study, in which the first half is diagnostic, and the second half is used for initiation and titration of noninvasive ventilation. This type of initiation is preferred by some clinicians[5] because it affords an objective assessment of sleep-disordered breathing and rapid optimization of ventilator settings. Also, ventilator settings can be optimized during sleep when respiratory control and upper airway resistance differs from the awake state.[6] On the other hand, use of a sleep laboratory may not be practical if none is available or if long delays are necessitated by crowded schedules. Further, patients with severe neuromuscular disease often have special needs that are poorly met in many sleep laboratories, and unless a caregiver can stay in the sleep laboratory with the patient, the experience may be unpleasant.

Other location options include the physician's office or the patient's home. If noninvasive ventilation is initiated in the physician's office, the home respiratory vendor should be contacted to provide equipment and a therapist for the office visit. The therapist assists in selecting and fitting the interface and adjusting the ventilator, while the physician makes certain that these are optimized, and also educates and motivates the patient. For initiation in the patient's home, a home respiratory vendor delivers equipment to the patient's home and a respiratory therapist provides education and training in noninvasive ventilation techniques. Because skill and experience with these techniques vary considerably between different home respiratory therapy companies and their therapists, home initiation should be used only when the therapist is highly skilled in the initiation of noninvasive ventilation.

Selection of Appropriate Personnel

The individuals identified to initiate noninvasive ventilation are critical to eventual success, and their importance in the process cannot be overemphasized. Their attitude and approach determine the patient's attitude, level of motivation, and willingness to cooperate. If they present themselves as skillful and knowledgeable clinicians, and appear confident that noninvasive ventilation will succeed, the chances of success will be much higher than if they have a negative attitude and appear to lack knowledge. Accordingly, any center using noninvasive ventilation should attempt to ascertain that clinicians administering it are trained and experienced in its proper application.

The above considerations are more important than the specific individuals who initiate NPPV, who will vary from institution to institution or from country to country. For acute applications in the United States, physicians are responsible for selecting appropriate patients, and usually, respiratory therapists, for initiation. Once the patient has started, nurses and therapists work together to assure that the patient successfully adapts. In countries lacking respiratory therapists, physicians and/or nurses are responsible for initiation. For chronic applications, the availability of home respiratory therapy services is key to eventual success. These permit frequent initial home visits so that problems are addressed promptly and assure that needed adjustments are made without delay. In countries lacking home respiratory therapy services, inpatient initiation is usually necessary for a long enough period of time to permit some adaptation.

Selection of a Ventilator

Characteristics of the various ventilators used for NPPV were discussed in Chapter 1. Clinicians must be knowledgeable regarding these characteristics, and also consider the patient's individual needs in choosing a ventilator. For acute applications, "bilevel" or critical care ventilators are usually chosen. For most patients, either type can be used successfully, and the choice is usually dictated by ventilator availability and clinician bias. Critical care ventilators may be preferred when sophisticated alarm or accurate monitoring capabilities are desired, or when patients have high inspiratory pressure or fraction of inspired oxygen (FiO$_2$) requirements. Bilevel pressure-limited ventilators may be preferred when better leak compensating abilities and fewer alarms are desired. These ventilators are also considerations if budgetary constraints limit the availability of critical care ventilators.

For chronic applications, simple to operate, lightweight ventilators are preferred. Bilevel ventilators have gained popularity for these reasons, particularly for patients requiring only nocturnal ventilatory assistance. For patients who require high inspiratory pressures or who have minimal spontaneous breathing capacity, portable volume-limited ventilators may be preferred because they have internal batteries and more sophisticated alarms. Of course, it is possible to obtain external batteries and alarms for bilevel ventilators. Portable volume-limited ventilators may also be preferred for patients with severe neuromuscular impairment because these devices permit breath "stacking," the retention of multiple tidal volumes to increase inspiratory volume and enhance cough flows.[7] It should also be recalled that some newer ventilators offer pressure-limited modes with sophisticated alarm and monitoring capabilities.

Selection of an Interface

Details related to the properties of different interfaces are provided in Chapter 1. The choice is based on patient characteristics, clinician preferences, availability, and cost considerations. For acute applications, nasal or oronasal masks are most often chosen, although some investigators begin with simple mouthpieces until patients have become accustomed to breathing with positive pressure. Either nasal or oronasal masks can be used successfully, but oronasal masks are chosen more often at many institutions in the United States. Nasal masks are preferred for claustrophobic patients or those who wish to be able to speak unimpeded. Nasal masks may also be preferable when airway secretions are more copious, because they permit unimpeded coughing and airway suctioning. Oronasal masks are preferred when patients have nasal obstruction or have excessive air leaks through the mouth despite use of a chin strap and coaching to keep the mouth shut. Regardless of the mask chosen, use of fitting gauges to avoid selection of a mask that is too large, and forehead spacers to minimize nasal ulcers, is encouraged.

For chronic respiratory failure, standard nasal masks are chosen most often, but gel masks, nasal "pillows," or minimasks may be preferred for enhanced patient comfort. Oronasal masks designed for noninvasive ventilation or mouthpieces may also be used, particularly if mouth leaking is a problem. Some patients with neuromuscular weakness who use NPPV on a nearly continuous basis may prefer to alternate between several different interfaces. In both acute and chronic settings, several mask sizes and styles may need to be tried to optimize fit and comfort. In the chronic setting, fit and comfort are overriding considerations and every effort should be made to optimize these, whereas in the acute setting, disposable masks are often used for brief periods of time, so cost is also an important concern. Clinicians are encouraged to have a variety of mask types and sizes readily available in the location where NPPV is to be initiated and, for this reason, some attach a "mask bag" containing a variety of mask types and sizes to ventilators used for noninvasive ventilation.

The Initiation Process

The steps for initiation are listed in Table 3, illustrated in Figure 1, and described in more detail below.

Table 3
10 Steps for Initiation of NPPV

---

1. Explain the process to the patient, select mask and ventilator.
2. Fit the mask, silence ventilator alarms (if present). Use of fitting gauge advised.
3. Initiate NPPV while holding the mask in place. Patient should hold mask, if possible.
4. Titrate inspiratory pressure (or volume) to patient comfort. Start low (6–8 cm H_2O), increase gradually (10–16 cm H_2O).
5. Secure the mask. Avoid excessive tightening of straps. Consider artificial skin.
6. Monitor O_2 sat, titrate FiO_2 for O_2 sat > 90%.
7. Titrate PEEP to minimize triger effort and increase O_2 sat.
8. Check for air leaks.
9. Avoid peak pressures > 20 cm H_2O.
10. Continue to coach and reassure, check patient frequently.

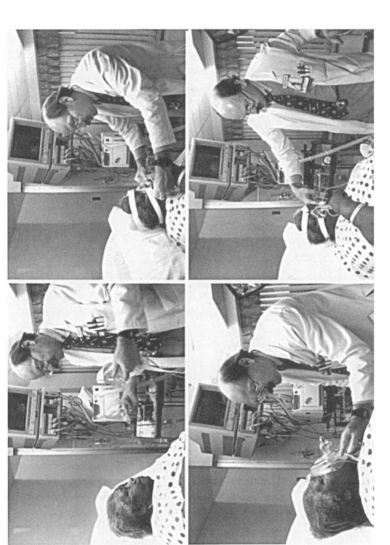

Figure 1. Some of the steps for initiating NPPV are shown. Upper left panel shows the patient sitting at 45° in bed while the process is explained to her. The lower left panel shows mask-fitting with an oronasal mask. The upper right panel shows the patient holding the mask in place while the straps are fastened. The lower right panel shows the clinician checking strap tension, assuring that 2 fingers can be inserted under the strap.

Explain the Process to the Patient

Once a ventilator and mask are chosen, successful implementation of NPPV depends, in large part, upon patient cooperation. The better the patient understands the therapy, the more likely it is that the patient will be motivated and compliant with NPPV. The goals of the therapy, the purpose of the interface, headgear, and ventilator, the steps to be taken during initiation, the expected response to NPPV and the potential problems, and all other aspects of the therapy should be explained to the patient. The clinician should also project an optimistic, confident attitude.

Fit the Mask and Silence Ventilator Alarms

Make sure the mask fit is optimal using a fitting gauge. During initiation of NPPV, ventilator alarms are distracting for the clinician and frightening for the patient. For this reason, ventilators that have few alarms or an alarm silence function are preferred for chronic applications unless the patient is dependent on continuous ventilation. In the acute setting, some clinicians use critical care ventilators with sophisticated alarms, but these should be silenced, if possible, during initiation.

Initiate NPPV While Holding the Interface in Place

A mask placed over the nose and/or mouth may be very frightening to a dyspneic patient. The patient should be allowed to acclimate to NPPV before strapping the mask on. It may be helpful to allow the patient to hold the mask (or other interface) in place initially before it is secured. Otherwise, the clinician should gently hold the mask in place before securing it with straps.

Titrate Inspiratory Pressure or Tidal Volume to Patient Comfort

Beginning with low settings (peak inspiratory pressure of 6–8 cm H_2O and expiratory pressure of 3–5 cm H_2O) helps the patient to comfortably acclimate to NPPV. Selection of an initial inspiratory pressure may be seen as a process of balancing the conflicting comfort goals (Figure 1). On one hand, the aim is to unload respiratory muscles and relieve respiratory discomfort, and this is achieved by rapidly increasing inspiratory pressure. On the other hand, raising inspiratory pressure may add to the discomfort of the mask and applied air pressure, and keeping this to a minimum will enhance patient tolerance. The "happy medium" can only be found by careful bedside titration performed by an experienced clinician working closely with the patient.

The inspiratory pressure is slowly increased (1–2 cm H_2O increments) and the patient's response is observed at each level. The clinician uses "eyeball" assessments of the patient's level of distress, maintains a dialogue with the patient, watches for reduced respiratory rate and elimination of accessory muscle use and abdominal paradox, and seeks good patient-ventilator synchrony. For some patients who are sensitive to air pressure, comfort is achieved only if the inspiratory pressure is lowered initially. After titration in the acute setting, typical initial inspiratory pressure is in the 10–16 cm H_2O range.

In the chronic setting, the process of pressure titration is essentially the same, but it is more important to avoid discomfort related to excessive air pressure than to relieve respiratory distress, which may even be absent in patients with neuromuscular disease. Accordingly, initial inspiratory pressures are lower than in the acute setting, typically 8–10 cm H_2O. The aim is to facilitate patient accommodation to the mask, particularly if nocturnal use during sleep is desired. Because patients are not acutely ill, the thinking is that there will be time to raise inspiratory pressures gradually over a period of weeks once the patient is more comfortable with the equipment. However, if the patient is rendered uncomfortable or frightened by excessive pressures initially, accommodation may be very difficult to achieve, and there may be no opportunity to increase inspiratory pressures later. In this sense, the selection of starting pressures may be seen as helping the patient over an initial "hurdle."

Some clinicians prefer volume-limited rather than pressure-limited ventilator modes. If a volume-limited mode is selected, the initiation process is essentially the same, except that the tidal volume rather than inspiratory pressure is titrated upward. Typically, initial tidal volumes are in the 10–15 mL/kg range, exceeding those chosen for invasive ventilation because of the need to compensate for leaks.[1]

The authors acknowledge that the above recommendations are based on clinical experience rather than objective scientific evidence.[8] Particularly in the acute setting, other clinicians prefer much higher initial pressures (i.e., 20 cm H_2O pressure support) to achieve rapid unloading of inspiratory muscles, and then titration of pressures downward if patients are intolerant.[9]

Secure the Mask

Once the patient is comfortable and breathing in synchrony with the ventilator, the headgear straps can be fastened. An excessively tight fit that makes NPPV more uncomfortable and increases the likelihood of complications can be avoided by making certain that one or two fingers can be slipped underneath the straps. For acute applications, artificial skin is routinely applied over the bridge of the nose or other sensitive areas to avoid nasal bridge ulcers. Some air leak under the mask seal usually will not compromise the effectiveness of NPPV, but the mask should be adjusted until excessive leaks are eliminated. Merely tightening straps more to eliminate leaks is ill-advised. Often, pulling the mask away from the face and re-seating the gasket will eliminate leaks without the need for further tightening. The patient should also be shown how to remove the mask when the straps are applied.

Monitor SpO_2 and Titrate FiO_2 to Achieve an O_2sat > 90%.

Oxygen is titrated into the mask or ventilator circuit; excessively high FiO_2 will raise oxygen saturation as measured by pulse oximetry (SpO_2) to a level that may potentially obscure detection of ventilatory difficulties. On the other hand, the ventilatory assistance usually prevents greater hypoventilation which otherwise may occur with O_2 supplementation in chronically hypercapnic patients. In patients with severe oxygen defects, ventilators with O_2 blenders that assure the delivery of precise O_2 concentrations may be preferred.

Titrate PEEP to Minimize Trigger Effort and Increase SpO_2

For patients with chronic obstructive pulmonary disease (COPD), positive end-expiratory pressure (PEEP) may be necessary to counterbalance auto-PEEP and improve triggering. In patients with alveolar pathology (e.g., congestive heart failure, pneumonia), PEEP may be useful to improve oxygenation. For chronic nocturnal applications, PEEP may be necessary to treat obstructive sleep apnea. PEEP is also useful to minimize rebreathing in bilevel ventilators. PEEP pressures of 4–5 cm H_2O are recommended for initiation. These are generally adequate to counterbalance auto-PEEP and minimize rebreathing. If triggering effort is excessive, breathing is asynchronous with the ventilator, or SpO_2 still too low, upward titration of PEEP (1–2 cm H_2O increments) may be tried.

Check for Air Leaks

Air leaks are universal during use of NPPV by virtue of its open circuit design. Pressure-limited ventilation can increase and prolong inspiratory air flow to compensate for small to moderate leaks, and tidal volumes can be raised to compensate during volume-limited ventilation. However, large leaks interfere with efficacy and can cause eye irritation, so these should be sought and corrected. Passing the fingers around the mask like a wand can detect leaks, and the mask can be reseated or the straps tightened to reduce them. Remember that leaks through the exhalation ports of bilevel ventilators are normal and are necessary for proper functioning.

Avoid Peak Pressures > 20 cm H_2O

Peak pressures > 20 cm H_2O are poorly tolerated and almost never needed, at least in the acute setting. Pressures above this level increase the likelihood of air leaks, discomfort due to sinus or ear pain and gastric insufflation, and they necessitate greater headgear strap tensions to control leaks. On the other hand, occasional patients with abnormal ventilatory mechanics, such as those with morbid obesity, may require high inspiratory pressures for adequate ventilation.

Continue to Coach and Reassure Patient

The need to closely observe the patient and make frequent adjustments to improve patient compliance during the initiation process cannot be overemphasized. Patients should be reassured and encouraged to coordinate their breathing pattern with the ventilator, keep the mask on, and breathe through their nose (when using a nasal mask). Prompts like "let the machine breathe for you" may be helpful. A positive, confident attitude on the part of practitioners can make the difference between success and failure. Pointing out to the patient that success means that endotracheal intubation will be avoided may also serve as a motivator.

Summary

Initiation of noninvasive ventilation is a simple process that requires attachment of a mask to the patient's face and to a ventilator, and selection of optimal ventilator settings. However, much more than invasive ventilation, success depends on patient motivation and cooperation. For this reason, initiation of noninvasive ventilation usually requires more clinician time than invasive ventilation, at least for the first few hours.[8] The clinician must choose an appropriate patient, find an acceptable location, optimize mask fit, and select a ventilator and optimal ventilator settings. This should be done in an efficient, but calm and relaxed manner, aimed at gaining the patient's confidence. Experience helps with this process, particularly when patients are having difficulty and readjustments are necessary. Success is dependent on the technical knowledge and skills of the practitioner and a willingness to work with the patient to optimize comfort and unloading of breathing muscles.

References

1. Leger P, Jennequin J, Gerard M, et al. Home positive pressure ventilation via nasal mask for patients with neuromuscular weakness or restrictive lung or chest wall deformities. Respir Care 1989;34:3-77.
2. Abboussouan LS, Khan SU, Meeker DP, et al. Effect of noninvasive positive pressure ventilation on survival in amyotrophic lateral sclerosis. Ann Intern Med 1997;127:450–453.
3. Plant PK, Owen JL, Elliott MW. Early use of noninvasive ventilation for acute exacerbations of chronic obstructive pulmonary disease on general respiratory wards: a multi-center randomized controlled trial. Lancet 2000;355:1931-1935.
4. Meecham Jones DJ, Paul EA, Jones PW. Nasal pressure support ventilation plus oxygen compared with oxygen therapy alone in hypercapnic COPD. Am J Respir Crit Care Med 1995;152:538-544.
5. Piper AJ, Sullivan CE. Effects of long-term nocturnal nasal ventilation on spontaneous breathing during sleep in neuromuscular and chest wall disorders. Eur Respir J 1996;9:1515-1522.
6. McNicholas WT. Impact of sleep in respiratory failure. Eur Respir J 1997;10:920-933.
7. Bach JR, Alba AS, Saporito LR. Intermittent positive pressure ventilation via the mouth as an alternative to tracheostomy for 257 ventilator users. Chest 1993;103:174-182.
8. Kramer N, Meyer TJ, Meharg J, et al: Randomized, prospective trial of noninvasive positive pressure ventilation in acute respiratory failure. Am J Respir Crit Care Med 1995;151:1799-1806.
9. Meduri GU, Abou-Shala N, Fox RC, et al. Noninvasive face mask mechanical ventilation in patients with acute hypercapnic respiratory failure. Chest 1991;100:445-454.

Chapter 3

Management and Monitoring of Noninvasive Positive Pressure Ventilation

Peter C. Gay, M.D., Nicholas S. Hill, M.D.

Introduction

Noninvasive ventilation offers an alternative to invasive positive pressure ventilation in the therapy of both acute and chronic forms of respiratory failure. Because of its potential to assist ventilation with greater comfort and less morbidity than invasive approaches, noninvasive positive pressure ventilation (NPPV) has seen rapidly increasing popularity in recent years. However, many centers have relatively little experience with its use and continue to underutilize it. Part of the problem may be related to a lack of familiarity with management and monitoring principles. Although many different types of ventilators can be used to deliver either invasive or noninvasive ventilation, there are fundamental differences in the way they are managed. Noninvasive ventilation, by its very design, sacrifices control over the airway, and there is no way to assure direct or leak-free access to the lower airways. In addition, noninvasive ventilation is largely dependent on patient cooperation for its success. For these reasons, management and monitoring of patients on NPPV is more patient-focused than with invasive ventilation. This chapter will discuss the approach to managing and monitoring adult patients after initiation of NPPV therapy, both in the acute and chronic settings. Pediatric management is discussed in Chapter 9.

Adaptation

Acute Applications

In the acute setting, the initiation phase is critically important to the eventual success of noninvasive ventilation. However, adaptation is

From *Noninvasive Positive Pressure Ventilation: Principles and Applications,* edited by Nicholas S. Hill. © 2001, Futura Publishing Company, Inc., Armonk, NY.

equally important if the initial success is to be sustained. This requires frequent checks on the patient status by knowledgeable physicians, nurses, and respiratory therapists. Clinicians must be sensitive to alterations in patient comfort, and frequent adjustments in ventilator settings, mask tension, or even mask type may be necessary. The clinician must also be alert to changes in the patient's respiratory or medical status that may indicate that weaning can be initiated or, less desirably, that a switch to invasive ventilation is necessary.

Ideally, patients with acute respiratory failure who are treated noninvasively should have reversible conditions that require only temporary ventilator assistance so that the duration of ventilator use ranges from hours to no more than a few days. Close attention to clinical parameters (as discussed below) helps to assure that ventilatory assistance is utilized optimally. Weaning should be undertaken as soon as the patient is ready, and intubation should not be needlessly delayed if the patient fails to respond favorably to noninvasive ventilation within a couple of hours.

Chronic Applications

For chronic applications of NPPV, adaptation is the most important aspect of success, and is even more important than initiation. This is because use is intended to be long-term, and successful adaptation requires that most patients learn to sleep with a foreign object strapped over the nose and/or mouth while pressurized air is blown through it. Not surprisingly, most patients encounter difficulty adapting and require frequent attention during the first several weeks.

During initiation, it is important to prepare patients for the adaptation process. They should be warned that adaptation is not easy and requires motivation and patience. They should be told that the process may take days, weeks, or even months, and that they should not give up easily. It may be helpful to compare the process with that of learning to play a musical instrument. Patients can appreciate that a musical instrument feels very foreign when it is first played, but with repeated practice sessions, one becomes expert at it. Likewise, adaptation to noninvasive ventilation requires repeated practice sessions before patients become comfortable and are able to sleep through the night.

During the adaptation process, home visits by a skilled respiratory therapist (usually employed by a durable medical equipment vendor) are highly desirable. The vendor delivers the noninvasive ventilator and other necessary equipment to the home, and reviews, in detail, the operation, application, and maintenance of the equipment. The patient is encouraged to begin using the equipment on the first night and to attempt to fall asleep. The patient is permitted to remove the mask if he/she awakens and wishes to do so. Forcing patients to suffer intolerable discomfort while attempting to adapt to noninvasive ventilation is counterproductive. Patients grow to dread use of the device and successful adaptation becomes impossible.

Early on, patients are also encouraged to use the ventilator for an hour or two while they are awake during the daytime, to facilitate familiarization. The home respiratory therapist should make several visits during this time to make certain that the apparatus is being properly used, and to make any adjustments or changes that are necessary to optimize comfort. This includes trying different interfaces or strap systems and adjusting pressures (or volumes). Initial pressures are usually relatively low to facilitate adaptation. If the patient complains of ear or sinus pain after the first few sessions, even lower pressures may be temporarily necessary. Usually, after the first week or 10 days, pressures (or volumes) can be gradually increased. As pressures exceed 10–12 cm H_2O and hours of use approach 4–6 hours per 24 hours, patients usually notice improved sleep and energy levels. When this threshold is reached, success becomes a virtual certainty as compliance is reinforced by the symptomatic improvement.

Interestingly, although patients are encouraged to use the ventilator during sleep, improvements in gas exchange will occur whether or not ventilator use is nocturnal.[1] Thus, patients who are having difficulty sleeping while using the device should be encouraged to increase hours of daytime use. Patients may find that reading or watching television helps to alleviate the tedium and boredom that they experience during daytime use of NPPV.

Communication between the patient, therapist, and physician is critical during the adaptation process. The physician is informed of problems as they arise and, in consultation with the therapist, suggests possible solutions based on prior experience. Using this approach in patients with restrictive thoracic disease who are motivated and persistent should be successful in the vast majority of properly selected patients. Despite equal or even greater efforts, success rates for patients with chronic obstructive pulmonary disease (COPD) tend to be lower than in those with restrictive disease.[2]

Monitoring

Appropriate monitoring is the key to the successful implementation of noninvasive ventilation. The specific parameters that are monitored correspond to the major goals of noninvasive ventilation (Table 1). In both acute and chronic settings, monitoring should occur at more frequent intervals initially, and then less often as the adaptation progresses. Successful monitoring requires close communication between physicians, nurses, and therapists so that problems are addressed quickly. The following section reviews basic principles of monitoring in both the acute and chronic settings as they apply to each of the main goals.

Monitoring in the Acute Setting

General Principles

Location. The best location to monitor patients using NPPV is determined by the patient's clinical status and need for continuous monitoring, rather than by arbitrary guidelines. Pragmatic considerations, such as unit and bed availability within a given institution, often override other considerations, but use of NPPV on general medical floors for patients at risk for sudden deterioration should be discouraged if high intensity beds are available. Often, NPPV is begun in the emergency department where the patient is placed in

Table 1

Goals and Monitoring of Noninvasive Ventilation in the Acute Setting

Goals	Monitored Variables
Subjective improvement	Comfort, respiratory distress
Improved gas exchange	Continuous pulse oximetry Arterial blood gases (as needed) Arterial line (optional)
Improved vital signs	Continuous electrocardiogram Respiratory and heart rates, blood pressure
Decreased work of breathing	Accessory muscle use Abdominal paradox
Good patient-ventilator synchrony	Triggering and cycling Delivered pressures and volumes
Minimizing complications	Mask fit—watch for sores of nasal bridge Air leaks Cough, secretions

a "code" or "trauma" room that permits continuous monitoring. Patients who remain at risk for sudden respiratory compromise are then transferred to an intensive care or respiratory step-down unit, where continuous noninvasive monitoring is available. It is important to continue ventilatory assistance during transfer. Patients can later be transferred to a regular medical or surgical floor once they have achieved stabilization of vital signs and gas exchange that is maintained for at least 20–30 minutes during unassisted breathing.

Personnel. The most important factors contributing to the success of NPPV are the familiarity of the patient's nurse and/or respiratory therapist with the technology, and their skill in helping the patient to successfully adapt. Their ability to respond to specific patient needs and to anticipate and ameliorate problems is a major determinant in obtaining good patient compliance. The general concept to apply when initiating and maintaining NPPV therapy is that a primary emphasis should be placed on achieving patient comfort. The more traditional focus of invasive ventilation on improving gas exchange becomes a secondary consideration. Institutions with the best success rates have a dedicated group of caregivers who are skilled in the use of NPPV, and who can respond to immediate changes at the bedside and make more frequent adjustments than would be considered routine with invasive ventilation.

Equipment. The equipment required for monitoring acutely ill patients using NPPV is the same as that commonly used for any form of respiratory compromise; continuous electrocardiography, pulse oximetry, vital signs with particular emphasis on respiratory and heart rates, and a qualitative assessment of patient-ventilator synchrony or tidal volume (Table 1). Many ventilators provide monitoring capabilities for tidal volume, minute volume, and mask pressures, and some can estimate air leak. However, these measures are less important than measures obtained from direct patient observation, because variable air leaks may render the ventilator measures inaccurate. Invasive monitoring is usually unnecessary, although an arterial line may be useful in patients with a tenuous hemodynamic status or the anticipated need for frequent arterial blood gas sampling.

Monitored Variables

Subjective Indexes and Bedside Observations. A primary objective of NPPV is to relieve the patient's respiratory distress while maintaining comfort levels acceptable to the patient. Hence, a simple "eyeball" test and brief patient interview are among the most valuable indicators.[3-5] It should be readily apparent whether or not the patient's sensation of dyspnea is reduced or if the patient is able to tolerate the discomfort associated with mask use and the positive pressure. Dyspnea scales are available to allow patients to quantify their sensation of dyspnea.[5] These may be helpful in assessing responses to therapy over time, but are of most use in research settings.

Numerous investigators have noted that early improvements (within 1–2 hr) in vital signs predict success of NPPV therapy.[4] Typically, initial respiratory rates that may be in the 30–40/min range fall to less than 30/min within the first hour or two, paralleled by reductions in heart rate (Figure 1).

Inspection of accessory muscle use and abdominal muscle paradox during inspiration should also reveal early improvements if NPPV is successfully applied, and this can be observed at the bedside. Further, patients with neurologic impairment will often improve with successful treatment, and a simple interview or use of mental status scales such as the Glasgow Coma score may be employed to monitor this therapeutic response. These bedside observations provide the practitioner with the most important feedback on the patient's response to therapy. By spending time with the patient during the initiation process and by making frequent bedside checks during the first few hours of adaption, medical personnel can promptly detect and treat potential problems while rapidly making adjustments to optimize comfort; thus, chances for success will be maximized.

Gas Exchange. Another major goal of NPPV is to ameliorate gas exchange defects. Accordingly, various measures of gas exchange are used during acute applications. The most commonly tracked measurement is continuous arterial oxygen saturation (SaO_2) which is best done by continuous pulse oximetry at the bedside (SpO_2) (Table 1). However, clinicians should not rely entirely on this measurement. Pulse oximetry requires accurate recordings of the arterial pulse which are prone to movement artifacts. Thus, values should not be relied upon unless the tracing is inspected for the stability and integrity of the pulse signal. Further, when patients are receiving O_2 supplementation, partial pressure of arterial carbon dioxide ($PaCO_2$) levels can rise substantially without any change in the SpO_2. This is of particular concern in patients with significant respiratory muscle weakness from neuromuscular disease who are prone to acute worsening of their

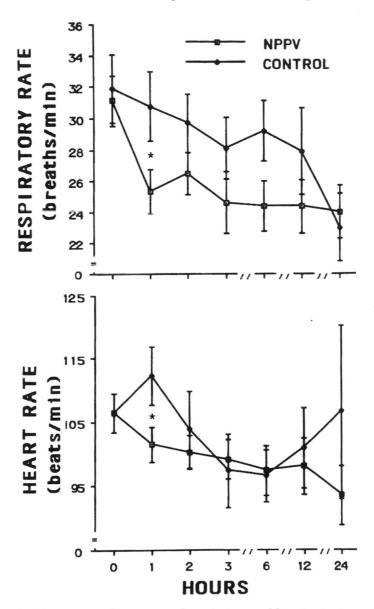

Figure 1. Time course of responses of respiratory and heart rates to noninvasive ventilation in patients treated with NPPV compared with controls treated conventionally. Respiratory rate drops promptly whereas the drop in heart rate is more gradual. *p<0.05 compared with control group. (From reference 6, with permission.)

hypercapnia if treated with oxygen alone.[6] Consequently, the baseline SpO_2 is best targeted near 90–92% so that improvements in SpO_2 more closely reflect changes in the patient's minute ventilation, synchrony with NPPV, or the other bedside observation targets previously noted.

Unfortunately, noninvasive measures of $PaCO_2$ have not been shown to be sufficiently accurate, so arterial blood gases remain the only clinically acceptable way of assessing $PaCO_2$ levels.[7] The use of arterial blood gases during NPPV treatment can also be useful to confirm the clinical impression of the patient's response and to assess the severity of respiratory acidosis. However, changes in blood gases may not necessarily occur as rapidly as relief of dyspnea or reduction in respiratory rate. Consequently, arterial blood gases are used sparingly, within the first hour or two of initiation to demonstrate some improvement (or exclude deterioration), and then as clinically indicated, particularly when there is concern that the patient is continuing to deteriorate. A typical time course for changes in pH and $PaCO_2$ and PaO_2 levels in a group of patients treated with NPPV is shown in Figure 2.

Failure of the $PaCO_2$ to improve during the first hour or two is not a concern as long as the patient is responding favorably in other ways. However, a further increase in $PaCO_2$ in concert with poor synchrony or sustained respiratory distress would constitute an indication for prompt intubation. For patients with chronic hypercapnia, further improvements in respiratory acidosis and $PaCO_2$ may occur over days, weeks, or longer. $PaCO_2$ need not be as rapidly or aggressively restored to baseline during acute episodes of exacerbation as compared to previously nonhypercapnic patients.[3,5]

Measures of Ventilator Function. In order to improve gas exchange with NPPV, adequate ventilatory assistance must be provided. Thus, monitoring of ventilator function is recommended although there is controversy over exactly which variables to monitor. One matter of debate is whether precise measurements of tidal and/or minute ventilation are necessary. Considering that there is almost always some air leak from the airway circuitry, mask, or mouth during NPPV, volume and flow measurements made by the ventilator are at best qualitative. Some studies have suggested that a tidal volume (V_T) > 7mL/kg or a minute volume (V_M) > 10 L/min during NPPV is more likely than lower volumes to be successful.[4] However, measuring the V_M was not predictive of the need for intubation, so it is unclear that additional clinical insight is truly gained by monitoring it. On the other hand, "critical care" ventilators are capable of accurate monitoring, and

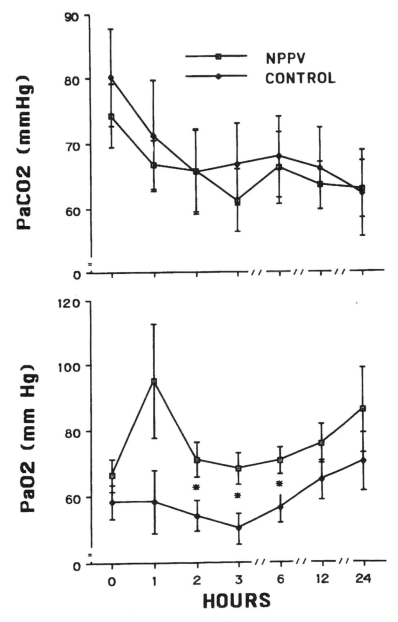

Figure 2. Time course of response of $PaCO_2$ and PaO_2 in patients treated with NPPV compared with controls. Oxygenation improves significantly more in NPPV-treated patients than in controls, accompanied by a gradual drop in $PaCO_2$. The control group experienced a similar drop in $PaCO_2$, mainly because patients in the control group who failed (2/3 of patients at 6 hr) were intubated and were no longer monitored. *$p<0.05$ compared with controls. (From reference 6, with permission.)

these measurements could be used to supplement bedside observations made regarding patient-ventilator synchrony, or to provide feedback on changes occurring with ventilator or equipment adjustments, or problems with air leak.

Other aspects of ventilator function that should be monitored include delivered inspiratory and expiratory pressures. The need to monitor these during volume-limited ventilation is obvious, but even during pressure-limited ventilation, there may be differences between actual pressures at the mask and preset pressures on the ventilator. The actual pressure may differ from the preset because of inaccuracy in ventilator settings, excessive air leak, or increased resistance in the ventilator circuit. Continuous tracings of flow, pressure, and volume may be quite helpful in assessing the impact of leaks and optimizing adjustments for comfort, but most often, these are not available.

Patient-Ventilator Synchrony. Another aspect of NPPV that is important to success and should be closely monitored is patient-ventilator synchrony. An important aim of NPPV in the acute setting is to unload the respiratory muscles, thereby preventing the development of frank respiratory muscle fatigue. In order to achieve this, the ventilator must provide increased positive pressure while the patient is inhaling, at approximately the same rate, without an excessive delay and not during exhalation. Accordingly, the patient must be able to coordinate beathing efforts with the ventilator, and the ventilator must be sensitive to the patient's breathing demands

Synchrony between the patient and ventilator is most easily evaluated by bedside observation. The patient triggers inspiratory flow from the ventilator with each breath, and the ventilator cycles easily into the expiratory phase when the patient ceases inspiring. This coordination of effort is usually quite obvious, and is signaled by comfort registered in the patient's facial expression and a reduction in sternocleidomastoid muscle activity.

Noninvasive monitoring techniques such as impedance plethysmography or magnetrometry are also helpful in establishing good synchrony, as shown in Figure 3, but these are mainly research tools and are not essential for usual clinical practice. Note in the figure that the pressure delivery tracing from the NPPV device and the excursion of the chest wall and abdomen (by inductance plethysmography) move in synchrony, indicating good coordination between the patient and ventilator. A poor synchrony response between patient and NPPV is shown in Figure 4. Here, there is discordance of the pressure and

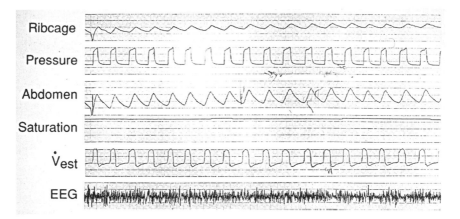

Figure 3. During this awake period, the patient's tidal volume is monitored by impedance plethysmography for rib cage and abdominal displacement. Mask pressure and estimated flow tracings ($\dot{V}_{est}$) are derived directly from the bilevel assist device external output. Notice the synchrony between pressure delivery by the device and breathing efforts of the patient.

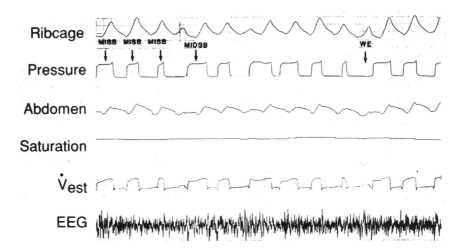

Figure 4. During light sleep, using the same recording technique as in Figure 3, the pressure and flow tracings become irregular as the device delivers breaths in a disrupted and ill-timed manner (MDISB, machine-initiated dyssynchronous breath). Note that the rib cage and abdominal excursions are reduced with dyssynchronous breathing. A reduced tidal volume may also occur if the machine fails to trigger and no assistance is given (WE, wasted effort).

plethysmographic tracings as the ventilator defaults to its mandatory backup rate and the breathing pattern is chaotic. The tidal volume during asynchrony is much lower than when the patient assists, so it is clear that good synchrony results in augmentation of V_T.

Failure to trigger may occur if patients who are using nasal masks breathe through their mouths, if large mask leaks are occurring, or if there is excessive intrinsic positive end-expiratory pressure (PEEPi). Careful monitoring of patient-ventilator synchrony allows for prompt corrective actions such as mask refitting, adjustment of inspiratory sensitivity or expiratory pressure settings, and coaching of the patient. These actions may greatly improve the level of actual minute ventilation that results during NPPV therapy. Large mask leaks may also interfere with synchrony during the expiratory phase of the respiratory cycle. Bilevel ventilators, in particular, may continue inspiratory pressure levels well into the expiratory phase.[8] The ability to limit inspiratory duration, as offered on newer bilevel ventilators, may help to control this problem.

Sleep Evaluation.   Although sleep is not routinely monitored in the acute setting, studies on patients treated in intensive or respiratory step-down units demonstrate severe disruption, correlated with the intensity of noise.[9] Sleep quality of patients receiving noninvasive ventilation is unlikely to be better than in those receiving invasive ventilation, and it may even be worse, considering that they frequently remove and replace the mask throughout the day and night. Unfortunately, other than attempting to minimize noise and disruptions, there is currently no intervention to improve sleep quality that would follow from the results of polysomnography, so it is not routinely done. Its main indications are to diagnose sleep-disordered breathing in those suspected of it (on the basis of a history of snoring or witnessed obstructive apneas), or to serve as a baseline in patients to be continued on long-term noninvasive ventilation after discharge from the hospital.

Avoiding Adverse Side Effects and Complications.   Another primary aim of the application of NPPV is to minimize the chances of adverse side effects or complications, and monitoring should be tailored to anticipate and minimize these. In this regard, monitoring for excessive air leaks is important. In contrast to invasive ventilation, noninvasive ventilation has no direct conduit to the lower airways, so leaks are inherent to its design. Leaks most commonly occur through the mouth (during nasal ventilation), or around the mask.

Some air leaking is not necessarily problematic; in fact, some ventilators such as bilevel devices have a built-in leak in the mask or ventilator circuitry that serves as an exhalation valve. However, excessive leak can interfere with the efficacy of noninvasive ventilation (see Chapter 10), and the amount and nature of air leak should be monitored. This can be achieved by bedside observation since gross air leaks are quite obvious, both visibly (as the lips or other upper airway structures vibrate) and audibly. More subtle leaks can be detected by tactile means, by circling the seal and lips with the fingers and feeling for a rush of air. When performing this maneuver, remember that some masks have small holes that are placed intentionally to serve as exhalation ports. During use of ventilators that monitor exhaled tidal volumes, leak can be estimated by subtracting exhaled tidal volume from the volume of air delivered during inspiration. Also, some portable pressure support ventilators generate estimates of the quantity of air leaked, although these estimates are imprecise.

Problems with mask discomfort, poor fit, and nasal pressure sores occur frequently during use of NPPV, as do mouth and nasal dryness and congestion. Patients should be checked frequently for these problems, so that they can be addressed promptly. Nasal redness should lead to adjustments to reduce pressure on the nose; many centers routinely place artificial skin over the skin of the nose to minimize the risk of ulceration.

Other problems inherent to noninvasive ventilation include the inability to directly suction the lower airways or to prevent aspiration. Accordingly, the patient's ability to clear secretions should be closely monitored, with consideration of intubation earlier rather than later if secretion retention occurs. Along these lines, aspiration is a concern, and earlier reports advised routine placement of a nasogastric tube with oronasal face mask ventilation.[4] However, aspiration does not appear to be a common event, and routine nasogastric tube placement is not currently recommended. Nonetheless, caution is warranted and practitioners should avoid NPPV in patients who are at high risk for aspiration and periodically reassess the patient's ability to protect the airway. Another aspect to monitor includes gastric insufflation, presumably related to the positive pressure being transmitted to the stomach.[10] Fortunately, this is rarely a major problem, probably because of the low inflation pressures used and the relatively high pressure at the lower esophageal sphincter. The management of the above problems will be discussed further in Chapter 10.

Weaning from Noninvasive Ventilation

Most patients treated for acute bouts of respiratory failure wean from NPPV within hours to a few days. The most often used weaning technique resembles T-piece weaning.[3,5] After vital signs and gas exchange have stabilized, the patient is permitted to temporarily discontinue mask ventilation and then resume if and when fatigue recurs. Periods off the ventilator are prolonged until, eventually, the patient no longer becomes distressed or fatigued during ventilator "rest" periods. In one study,[5] patients used the ventilator for an average of 20 of the first 24 hours, and 14 of the second 24 hours if they continued use. An alternative approach to weaning is to gradually lower inspiratory pressure levels as is done with pressure support weaning during invasive ventilation. No study has compared different approaches with weaning from NPPV, and many patients take an active role in weaning as they remove the masks themselves.

Occasional patients recovering from bouts of acute respiratory failure may continue to use NPPV nocturnally. Although no guidelines have been established for the selection of these patients, they are usually patients with severely impaired ventilatory function who remain severely hypercarbic despite NPPV therapy. A sleep evaluation may be useful in these patients before discharge to the home, to exclude sleep-disordered breathing and to assure adequate nocturnal oxygenation.

Monitoring in the Chronic Setting

General Principles

Location.   As opposed to the acute setting, monitoring by clinicians in the chronic setting is intermittent, and after successful adaptation, may occur quite infrequently, as few as 2 or 3 times yearly. Most monitoring takes place in the home or chronic care facility. The ability to monitor in the home depends on the competency of home caregivers and the availability of visiting nurses or home respiratory therapists to visit the patient. Patients are also evaluated periodically in physician's offices, sleep laboratories, or inpatient units, depending on clinical needs.

Personnel.   These include the patient's family, personal caregivers, visiting nurses, and respiratory therapists from the home respiratory care vendor. These individuals address questions and report problems to the physician. Visits to the physician's office or hospital are arranged periodically, as clinically indicated.

Equipment. Monitoring of symptoms and signs is key to the follow-up of patients receiving long-term noninvasive ventilation (Table 2). Occasional arterial blood gases and sleep monitoring using oximetry or portable multichannel recorders is helpful in confirming that gas exchange is being adequately supported. Full polysomnography may be useful during initial assessment of initiation of NPPV, but its routine role in subsequent monitoring has not been established.

Follow-Up Interval. The frequency of monitoring for patients using long-term noninvasive ventilation depends on the underlying disorder, duration of NPPV use, ease of adaptation, and whether problems arise. Ideally, patients should be seen weekly in the home by the home respiratory therapist for the first several weeks after initiation. This allows for proper adjustment of mask fit and gradual upward titration of

Table 2
Goals and Monitoring of Noninvasive Ventilation in the Chronic Setting

Goals	Monitoring Variables
Alleviate symptoms	Fatigue
	Somnolence
	Morning headache
	Dyspnea
Improve signs of cor pulmonale	Pedal edema
	Neck vein distension
	Heart sounds
Improve gas exchange	Arterial blood gases (occasional)
	SPO_2, transcutaneous or end-tidal
	PCO_2 (spot checks)
Improve sleep quality	Nocturnal oximetry
	Multichannel reading
	Polysomnography
Improve health status, functional capacity	Health status questionnaires
	6-minute walk test
Maintain pulmonary function	Spirometry
	Lung volumes
	Peak expiratory flow
Improve survival	Continued follow-up

pressures. These visits also reinforce patient use of NPPV and probably improve patient compliance compared with less frequent follow-up intervals, although this has not been established in controlled studies. If patients have problems, the therapist can notify the physician and discuss possible solutions. The therapist can also check the timer on the ventilator to assess patient use. Although once weekly visits are adequate for most patients, the frequency of therapist visits should be tailored to patient need. Unfortunately, reimbursement limitations imposed by the Health Care Financing Agency (HCFA) have made it difficult for home vendors to provide services to patients who are having problems adapting.

A physician visit scheduled within the first 3–4 weeks is helpful to discuss progress and enhance motivation. This also permits assessment of symptoms and detailed questioning regarding problems that may be encountered. Arterial blood gases are generally not helpful unless the patient is using the ventilator for at least 4–6 hours per 24 hours, or unless symptoms suggest worsening. Patients who are not yet experiencing symptomatic improvement are at risk of discontinuing therapy and should be strongly encouraged to persevere. A second physician's visit should be scheduled at the 2–3 month time point, which is when some third party payers now require a physician assessment to certify adequate compliance and effectiveness. Afterwards, follow-up visits are scheduled as needed, but stable patients who have adapted successfully and who are not experiencing problems may be seen as infrequently as once or twice yearly. Patients with more rapidly progressive diseases such as motor neuron disease are seen more often.

Monitored Variables

Alleviation of Signs and Symptoms. A major aim of long-term noninvasive ventilation is to alleviate symptoms related to hypoventilation and impaired sleep. These include symptoms attributable to sleep disruption, such as fatigue and daytime hypersomnolence, and to nocturnal CO_2 retention, such as morning headache. Hence, monitoring should assess whether or not these symptoms are improved. Sleepiness scales, such as the Epworth Sleepiness Score[11] may be used to monitor responses, as may questionnaires to assess health status. The latter are more often used as research tools, however, and do not necessarily add to a simple patient interview by the therapist or physician. Monitoring physical findings is also important during use of noninvasive ventilation. Heart rate may drop, and signs of cor pulmonale, including neck vein distention, an increase in the pulmonic component of the second heart sound, liver enlargement, and peripheral edema may resolve.

When noninvasive ventilation is successful, symptoms and signs invariably improve, sometimes in dramatic fashion. This improvement also serves as a strong reinforcement for the patient to continue use. In contrast to symptoms attributable to hypoventilation or poor sleep quality, the resolution of dyspnea is not so consistent. Patients with severe neuromuscular disease may have no sensation of dyspnea, even in the face of severe respiratory failure. Dyspnea is more consistently found in patients with chest wall deformity or obstructive lung disease. However, institution of noninvasive ventilation may not improve dyspnea in these patients, unless its use is associated with improvements in spontaneous ventilatory capacity.

Gas Exchange.　Arterial blood gases have long been the gold standard for the assessment of pulmonary gas exchange. Results vary from laboratory to laboratory with proficiency standards for $PaCO_2$ and PaO_2, as determined by the College of American Pathologists, of $\pm$ 3 torr and $\pm$ 7.5%, respectively.[12] For monitoring purposes in patients using noninvasive ventilation, daytime arterial blood gases are routinely used as the main indicator of improvement in gas exchange. Blood gases are usually checked 2–6 weeks after initiation of noninvasive ventilation when patients are using the ventilator at least 4–6 hours per 24 hours, and then periodically thereafter. $PaCO_2$ invariably falls and PaO_2 rises when noninvasive ventilation is used successfully in hypoventilating patients with neuromuscular disease or chest wall deformity. A lack of improvement should trigger additional therapeutic efforts or diagnostic studies to determine the reason for failure.

The ideal target value for daytime $PaCO_2$ during noninvasive ventilation has not been established, but normalization of daytime $PaCO_2$ is neither necessary nor even desirable. In the authors experience, patients experience symptomatic relief and resolution of signs of cor pulmonale even when daytime spontaneous $PaCO_2$ cannot be lowered below the mid 50s mm Hg or even low 60s mm Hg. The patient's ventilatory impairment may make it difficult to lower daytime $PaCO_2$ below this level without an increase in inspiratory pressure or a prolongation of the duration of ventilator use that is unacceptable to the patient. In addition, maintenance of a normal $PaCO_2$ requires a higher level of alveolar ventilation than an elevated $PaCO_2$ and would be potentially more fatiguing to the patient. Thus, the ideal $PaCO_2$ level probably differs from patient to patient and in the same patient over time, depending on the severity of the ventilatory impairment and the level of hypercapnia at which symptoms worsen.

Although arterial blood gas monitoring provides the most accurate measure of $PaCO_2$, it is invasive and requires ready access to a blood gas machine, so some clinicians advocate the use of noninvasive measures of gas exchange as a way to monitor responses to noninvasive ventilation.[13] Pulse oximetry is adequate to assure a desired level of oxygenation, but even when oxygen saturation is normal, CO_2 retention may be substantial. Unfortunately, noninvasive measures of CO_2 have not proven to be sufficiently accurate to replace blood gases. End-tidal CO_2 measurements can be misleading during noninvasive ventilation, because of bias flow with some ventilator types and air leaks that may lead to underestimation of the actual CO_2 level. Devices that measure transcutaneous CO_2 tension have been hampered by the need for heated transducers and frequent calibration. In addition, although recent studies suggest that the technology is improving,[14] measurements have been imprecise and response times slow.[7]

On the other hand, noninvasive measures of gas exchange may be useful for nocturnal monitoring. Continuous nocturnal oximetry has been used to assess responses to nasal CPAP in patients with obstructive sleep apnea,[15] and likewise, it provides an accurate assessment of the adequacy of oxygenation during noninvasive ventilation. Unfortunately, it may not accurately reflect changes in $PaCO_2$, particularly during use of supplemental oxygen. Transcutaneous CO_2 monitoring during sleep can be helpful in establishing trends and confirming the adequacy of ventilation over many minutes or hours. Unfortunately, the response time is too slow to detect transient episodes of hypoventilation. Also, patient movements that cause alterations in transducer position may lead to upward or downward drifting in the recorder signal and the need for frequent recalibration. These problems limit the utility of transcutaneous CO_2 recording in busy clinical sleep laboratories, so it has been used mainly as a research technique.

Sleep Evaluation. Sleep-disordered breathing is an important component of chronic respiratory failure[16] and occasional sleep monitoring for follow-up of noninvasive ventilation has been advocated by most authorities.[17,18] However, the specific technique that should be used for sleep monitoring is a matter of debate. Full facility-based polysomnography remains the gold standard, but it is expensive, may be difficult to arrange on short notice, and may be uncomfortable for neuromuscular patients. Simple nocturnal oximetry may suffice as a screening technique to assure adequacy of gas exchange. If abnormalities are detected, then more sophisticated monitoring must be done to identify the cause of the abnormalities. For this purpose, multichannel recorders that monitor nasal air flow, chest wall impedance, the electrocardiogram, and oximetry may be quite useful for home monitoring. These allow assessment of apneic or hypopneic episodes of an obstructive or central nature. However, unattended home monitoring is subject to artifacts related to positional changes or electrode migration and must be interpreted with caution.

The only way to accurately assess effects of noninvasive ventilation on sleep quality and duration is to perform a full polysomnogram including electroencephalography. However, unless it is demonstrated that such detailed monitoring is necessary to optimize the efficacy of noninvasive ventilation, it is difficult to recommend that full polysomnography be included as part of routine monitoring. From a pragmatic viewpoint, clinicians can probably assume that if symptoms such as fatigue and daytime hypersomnolence resolve with noninvasive ventilation, sleep quality has improved. Furthermore, if nocturnal oximetry or portable multichannel recordings performed in the home show adequate support of gas exchange and amelioration of hypopneas, it is unlikely that findings from full polysomnography will substantially alter the management approach.

On the other hand, studies using full polysomnography have demonstrated the occurrence of frequent arousals associated with air leak through the mouth despite adequate support of gas exchange.[19] If techniques are developed that can successfully reduce air leak and associated arousals, then full polysomnography to assess the frequency of arousals could be useful. Pending more definitive information, the current recommendation would be to monitor overnight oximetry 2–6 weeks after initiation of NPPV, when the patient is using the device at least 4–6 hours nightly. If frequent or sustained desaturations are detected, then more sophisticated monitoring is indicated to decipher the cause, including polysomnography. Figure 4 provides an example of how polysomnography may be helpful in detecting asynchronous breathing. Also, repeat oximetry is indicated if symptoms deteriorate after successful initial adaptation to noninvasive ventilation.

Health Status and Functional Capacity.   A goal of any major and costly therapeutic intervention in patients with chronic lung disease should be an improvement in overall health status (sometimes referred to as quality of life). Absent this improvement, the value of the intervention should be seriously questioned. Although most studies have not examined this variable, a few have shown improvement, after noninvasive ventilation, in validated questionnaires such as the St. George's Respiratory Questionnaire.[20,21] Although many pulmonary rehabilitation programs are including such questionnaires, they also include general health status assessments, such as the SF-36,[22] as a routine part of their follow-up. Although such assessments are not essential for the individual practitioner who treats patients with noninvasive ventilation, they may be helpful. At the least, patients should be routinely queried about their overall level of functioning.

Another aim of noninvasive ventilation is to improve functional status. However, improvements in respiratory or other muscle strength and endurance are not consistently seen. Moreover, many patients receiving noninvasive ventilation have severe neuromuscular disease, and the expectation of substantial improvements in functional capacity among these patients would be unrealistic. Thus, it is not surprising that improvements in overall functional capacity as determined by treadmill walking time or the 6-minute walk distance have been diffi-cult to demonstrate.[23,24] These measures are mainly of interest in re-search studies and need not be done on a routine basis. Nonetheless, questioning patients about functional status is a routine part of periodic outpatient follow-up.

Pulmonary Function. The frequency of monitoring of pulmonary function depends on the anticipated rapidity of progression of the underlying respiratory impairment and changes in the patient's clinical state. At the very least, spirometry should be monitored once or twice yearly in patients with progressive neuromuscular diseases, so that the rate of progression and severity of dysfunction can be ascertained. The spirogram and lung volumes should be measured prior to initiation, but the latter need not be repeated frequently unless there are concerns about changes in the patient's lung or chest wall compliance. A decline in the vital capacity to below 40–50% of the predicted value (1–1.5 L) has been shown to correlate with CO_2 retention in patients with neuromuscular disease,[25] and further declines below this level after initiation of noninvasive ventilation may indicate the need for increasing hours of ventilator use.

Reductions in maximal inspiratory pressure (MIP) and maximal ex-piratory pressure (MEP) have also been shown to correlate with the onset of respiratory failure and are commonly measured during follow-up.[25]

Retention of CO_2 is rare if MIP is greater than 50% of the predicted value, but common if MIP is below 33% of the predicted value. The accuracy of MIP and MEP measurements is less than that for vital capacity, however, and combining these measures with vital capacity has not been shown to add any prognostic information. The peak expiratory flow or "peak cough flow" measured using a simple hand-held peak flow meter is also a useful measurement in patients with severe neuromuscular impairment, serving as an objective measure of coughing ability.[26] Peak cough flows exceeding 3 L/sec with or without cough assisting maneuvers have been shown to correlate with successful removal of tracheostomies in patients with chronic respiratory failure.[26]

Monitoring for Adverse Side Effects and Complications. Another important aim of the use of NPPV is to administer it safely and to avoid complications (see Chapter 10). In order to achieve this aim, practitioners must have knowledge regarding the occurrence of adverse side effects and complications, and of how to avoid and treat them. Perhaps the most important step in avoiding complications is to select appropriate recipients of noninvasive ventilation. If patients have intact upper airway function and are able to cooperate, success rates will be much higher than if these attributes are lacking.

Nonetheless, certain adverse effects should be anticipated and promptly addressed if success rates are to be maximized. In general, side effects and complications include those associated with the mask and air pressure or flow from the ventilator, failure to improve ventilation, and other major complications.[10] During adaptation in the chronic setting, these problems arise frequently and should be identified and promptly addressed by the respiratory therapist and physician working in tandem. The therapist should visit the patient intermittently during the first several weeks, making adjustments in the mask, headgear, and ventilator settings as needed, and the patient should visit the physician's office periodically to be interviewed and examined. The patient should be queried about difficulties with adaptation and hours of use. The physician should encourage the patient to gradually increase hours of use and should contact the therapist with suggestions about adjustments to enhance adaptation.

Summary

Proper monitoring of NPPV use is critically important in maximizing the chances for success, whether in the acute or chronic setting.

The practitioner must have a clear idea of the goals, a knowledge of the equipment, the variables to be monitored and anticipated responses, and, ideally, experience with problems that are likely to be encountered. In the acute setting, the aim is to achieve rapid acceptance with alleviation of respiratory distress and gas exchange abnormalities. Accordingly, monitoring focuses on subjective responses, vital signs, and gas exchange. In the chronic setting, gas exchange is also important, but patient comfort is paramount for successful adaptation. For this reason, more attention is paid to acceptance of the interface and avoiding discomfort related to the use of excessive air pressure early in the process. With attention to these monitoring principles, practitioners can optimize patient tolerance and achieve success in the majority of patients.

References

1. Schonhofer B, Geibel M, Sonneborn M, et al. Daytime mechanical ventilation in chronic respiratory insufficiency. Eur Respir J 1997;10:2840-2846.
2. Criner GJ, Brennan K, Travaline JM, Kreimer D. Efficacy and compliance with noninvasive positive pressure ventilation in patients with chronic respiratory failure. Chest 1999;116:665-667.
3. Brochard L, Isabey D, Piquet J, et al. Reversal of acute exacerbations of chronic obstructive lung disease by inspiratory assistance with a face mask. N Engl J Med 1990;323(22):1523-1530.
4. Meduri GU, Abou-Shala N, Fox RC, et al. Noninvasive face mask mechanical ventilation in patients with acute hypercapnic respiratory failure. Chest 1991;100(2):445-454.
5. Kramer N, Meyer TJ, Meharg J, et al. Randomized, prospective trial of noninvasive positive pressure ventilation in acute respiratory failure. Am J Respir Crit Care Med 1995;151(6):1799-1806.
6. Gay PC, Edmonds LC. Severe hypercapnia after low-flow oxygen therapy in patients with neuromuscular disease and diaphragmatic dysfunction. Mayo Clin Proc 1995;70(4):327-330.
7. Sanders MH, Kern NB, Costantino JP, et al: Accuracy of end-tidal and transcutaneous PCO_2 monitoring during sleep. Chest 1994;106:472-483.
8. Calderini E, Confalonieri M, Puccio PG, et al. Patient-ventilator asynchrony during noninvasive ventilation: the role of expiratory trigger. Intensive Care Med 1999;25:662-667.
9. Meyer TJ, Eveloff SE, Bauer MS, et al. Adverse environmental conditions in the respiratory and medical intensive care unit settings. Chest 1994;105:1211-1216.
10. Hill NS. Complications of noninvasive positive pressure ventilation. Respir Care 1997;42:432-442.
11. Johns MW. A new method for measuring daytime sleepiness: the Epworth Sleepiness Scale. Sleep 1991;14:540-545.

12. Shapiro BA. Evaluation of blood gas monitors: performance criteria, clinical impact, and cost/benefit. Crit Care Med 1994;22:546-548.
13. 1Bach JR, Alba AS, Saporito LR. Intermittent positive pressure ventilation via the mouth as an alternative to tracheostomy for 257 ventilator users. Chest 1993;103:174-182.
14. Janssens JP, Howarth-Frey C, Chevrolet JC, et al. Transcutaneous PCO_2 to monitor noninvasive mechanical ventilation in adults: assessment of a new transcutaneous PCO_2 device. Chest 1998;113:786-773.
15. Tobert DG, Gay PC. New directions for pulse oximetry in sleep disorders. Mayo Clin Proc 1995;70(6):591-592.
16. McNicholas WT. Impact of sleep in respiratory failure. Eur Respir J 1997;10:920-933.
17. Gay PC, Patel AM, Viggiano RW, Hubmayr RD. Nocturnal nasal ventilation for treatment of patients with hypercapnic respiratory failure. Mayo Clin Proc 1991;66(7):695-703.
18. Piper AJ, Sullivan CE. Effects of long-term nocturnal nasal ventilation on spontaneous breathing during sleep in neuromuscular and chest wall disorders. Eur Respir J 1996;19:1515-1522.
19. Meyer TJ, Pressman MR, Benditt J, et al. Air leaking through the mouth during nocturnal nasal ventilation: effect on sleep quality. Sleep 1997;20:561-569.
20. Elliott MW, Simonds AK, Carroll MP, et al. Domiciliary nocturnal nasal intermittent positive pressure ventilation in hypercapnic respiratory failure due to chronic obstructive lung disease effects on sleep and quality of life. Thorax 1992;47(5):342-348.
21. Meecham Jones DJ, Paul EA, Jones PW. Nasal pressure support ventilation plus oxygen compared with oxygen therapy along in hypercapnic COPD. Am J Respir Crit Care Med 1995;152:538-544.
22. Mahler DA, Mackowiak JI. Evaluation of short-form 36-item questionnaire to measure health-related quality of life in patients with COPD. Chest 1995;107:1585-1589.
23. Strumpf DA, Millman RP, Carlisle CC, et al. Nocturnal positive-pressure ventilation via nasal mask in patients with severe chronic obstructive pulmonary disease. Am Rev Respir Dis 1991;144:1234-1239.
24. Guyett GH, Sullivan MJ, Thompson PJ, et al. The 6-minute walk: a new measure of exercise capacity in patients with chronic heart failure. Can Med Assoc J 1985;132:919-923.
25. Braun NMT, Arora NS, Rochester DF. Respiratory muscle and pulmonary function in polymyositis and other proximal myopathies. Thorax 1983;38:616-623.
26. Bach JR, Saporito LR. Criteria for extubation and tracheostomy tube removal for patients with ventilatory failure: a different approach to weaning. Chest 1996;110:1566-1571.

Chapter 4

Noninvasive Mechanical Ventilation for Acute Exacerbations of Chronic Obstructive Pulmonary Disease

Nicolino Ambrosino, M.D., Michele Vitacca, M.D.

Introduction

Mechanical ventilation is indicated in the treatment of acute exacerbations of chronic obstructive pulmonary disease (COPD) when conservative therapy fails. Until recently, endotracheal intubation was considered the preferred route for mechanical ventilation. However, use of invasive mechanical ventilation is associated with complications that may be avoided by noninvasive methods. Noninvasive positive pressure ventilation (NPPV) via a face or a nasal mask has been used increasingly for this purpose.

Success with NPPV in acute COPD exacerbations has been reported in 51–91% of cases and is predicted by less severely abnormal baseline clinical and gas exchange parameters, and less severe levels of acidosis than in failures. Therefore, NPPV should be used in selected patients. The following reviews the evidence supporting the use of NPPV in COPD exacerbations, discusses predictors of successful therapy, and makes recommendations for selection of appropriate candidates for NPPV therapy.

Rationale for the Use of Noninvasive Ventilation

For decades, the mechanical ventilatory mode of first choice for acute respiratory failure in most intensive care units (ICUs) worldwide has been positive pressure ventilation administered via a translaryngeal endotracheal intubation, or when respiratory failure is prolonged, via a tracheostomy tube.[1,2] These techniques expose the patient to the

From *Noninvasive Positive Pressure Ventilation: Principles and Applications,* edited by Nicholas S. Hill. © 2001, Futura Publishing Company, Inc., Armonk, NY.

risk of a variety of complications that arise during the endotracheal intubation or tracheostomy procedure, during the course of mechanical ventilation, or after removal of the tube (Table 1).[3] Endotracheal intubation also provides a direct conduit to the lung for foreign material and increases the risk of nosocomial pneumonia and sinusitis. It interferes with eating and speech, contributing to the patient's psychological stress, and requires use of sedation to maintain comfort, often delaying the weaning process.

In selected patients, noninvasive ventilation can provide a number of advantages over invasive ventilation and offer a similar degree of efficacy. By preserving upper airway function including cough and swallowing, leaving the oronasal humidification mechanism intact, and enhancing patient comfort and thereby reducing the need for sedation, noninvasive ventilation avoids many of the complications associated with invasive mechanical ventilation (Table 2). In so doing, NPPV

Table 1
Complications Associated with Intubation and Mechanical Ventilation[3]

Prolonged and delayed intubation
    Cardiac arrest,
    Generalized seizures
    Gastric distension
Self-extubation
Trauma and mechanical dysfunction
    Cuff leaks
    Injury to the pharynx, larynx, and trachea
        Ulceration
        Edema
        Hemorrhage
        Stenosis
    Loss of voice and ability to eat normally
Respiratory muscle dysfunction and atrophy
Nosocomial infections
    Sinusitis
    Ventilator-associated pneumonia
Decrease in cardiac output
Barotrauma and ventilator-induced lung injury
Increased work of breathing
Prolonged weaning
Complications associated with monitoring
    Pulmonary artery catheter complications

Table 2
Advantages of Noninvasive Ventilation

- Avoids trauma of endotracheal intubation.
- Airway defenses left intact.
- Enhanced comfort; ventilatory assistance may be interrupted.
- Normal swallowing, feeding, speech.
- Physiologic air warming and humidification.
- Physiologic cough.
- Less sedation, easier weaning.
- Endotracheal intubation still possible if necessary.

has the potential of reducing patient morbidity and mortality, and by facilitating the weaning process from mechanical ventilation, reducing health care costs.

Physiologic Effects of NPPV in COPD Patients

Pathophysiologic Considerations

In order to better understand the physiologic effects of NPPV and how best to provide ventilatory support, an appreciation of the unique pathophysiologic defects of severe COPD is helpful. Most patients with severe COPD have a combination of pathologic abnormalities consisting of greater or lesser degrees of emphysema, chronic bronchitis, and bronchospasm. Before mechanical ventilation is contemplated, medical therapy to treat the potentially reversible inflammatory and bronchospastic components should be optimized, but many patients are still left with severe, largely irreversible disease consisting of a substantial emphysematous component. These patients have increased lung compliance and during expiration, their small airways tend to collapse and limit expiratory flow, both related to the destruction of lung parenchyma and the loss of elastic structures.

The consequence of the increased lung compliance and expiratory flow limitation is hyperinflation, with flattening of the diaphragm and recruitment of accessory muscles of breathing. These adaptations are necessary to maintain adequate ventilation, but they greatly reduce the efficiency of breathing, and increase its energy cost. Even under baseline conditions, these patients often are breathing so inefficiently that they are close to the point of developing respiratory muscle fatigue, and a relatively minor increase in demand, such as that imposed by mild exercise, may push them beyond that point.

During a COPD exacerbation, expiratory resistance often rises related to inflammation and bronchospasm, and as with exercise, the small increase in breathing load may precipitate respiratory muscle fatigue. In an effort to maintain expiratory air flow, the patient further hyperinflates the lungs and worsens ventilatory efficiency. Respiratory rate increases, limiting the time available for expiration, and contributing to auto-positive end-expiratory pressure (auto-PEEP), the positive pressure remaining in alveoli at end-expiration related to incomplete emptying. Because the alveolar pressure must be reduced to subatmospheric levels to initiate the next breath, the auto-PEEP further increases the inspiratory load, and a downward cycle toward respiratory muscle fatigue and failure ensues.

Actions of NPPV

NPPV can be used to interrupt the downward spiral. Because the insult that precipitates the respiratory crisis is often a mild one superimposed on a severe underlying pathophysiologic defect, relatively small amounts of ventilatory assistance can restore equilibrium. In this regard, NPPV is used as a form of *partial* ventilatory assistance, serving as a "crutch" to assist the patient until medical therapies and time can reduce the airway resistance, and the patient can resume unassisted breathing.

Studies both in obstructive and in restrictive patients[4,5] demonstrate that when patients coordinate their breathing with the noninvasive ventilator, whether delivered in the assist/control (A/C) or pressure support ventilation (PSV) modes, inspiratory muscle work falls significantly. In stable COPD patients, NPPV increases minute ventilation and tidal volume, and reduces transdiaphragmatic pressure and breathing frequency while improving gas exchange.[5] In addition, imposition of external positive end-expiratory pressure (PEEPe) enhances the inspiratory assistance provided by inspiratory pressure support alone. This occurs because of the counterbalancing effect of PEEPe on auto-PEEP, reducing the drop in alveolar pressure necessary to initiate the next breath and thereby lowering the inspiratory threshold.[5,6] In summary, COPD exacerbations increase the inspiratory muscle load, and by providing inspiratory assistance as well as expiratory pressure,

NPPV forestalls the development of respiratory muscle fatigue and failure in patients with acute on chronic respiratory impairments.

Evidence for Efficacy

Success Rate

A review of the literature since 1989 shows that use of NPPV in acute respiratory failure has been reported in many studies comprising a total of more than 700 patients, most of whom had COPD.[7-11] Only 5 studies were randomized, controlled trials (Table 3),[12-16] whereas most were retrospective case series or used historical controls. Success among all the studies, defined as tolerance of NPPV by the patient with improvement in gas exchange and avoidance of endotracheal intubation, was reported in 51–93% of cases. This wide range can be explained by the fact that the severity of acute respiratory failure, as assessed by the level of respiratory acidosis, differed widely between the studies.[7-16]

The first controlled study of NPPV in acute COPD exacerbations randomized 30 patients to use nasal masks and volume-limited ventilation and 30 to serve as controls.[12] NPPV patients had more rapid reductions in $PaCO_2$ and dyspnea scores, and NPPV reduced mortality rate from 30% in controls to 9%. The reduction in mortality rate was not statistically significant, however, until 4 NPPV patients, 2 of whom died, were excluded from the analysis because they never actually received NPPV. It is also notable that very few of the control patients received any form of mechanical ventilation, so this study can also be viewed as a trial of NPPV in patients who had COPD exacerbations and were not intubated.

Table 3
Time Spent in ICU/Hospital Stay (Mean days±SD)

Reference	Control	NPPV
Bott et al.[12]	9	9
Brochard et al.[14]	35 ± 33	23(±17)*
Kramer et al.[13]	17 ± 3	15 ± 3
Celikel et al.[15]	13 ± 2	10 ± 2*
Barbe et al.[16]	11 ± 2	11 ± 2

*p < 0.05 for significant differences.

In a subsequent trial, Kramer et al.[13] used nasal ventilation with a BiPAP™ (Respironics, Inc., Murrysville, PA) device in 31 patients randomized to receive NPPV or conventional therapy. They observed more rapid improvements in respiratory rate and $PaCO_2$ patients, and a significant reduction in the need for intubation (26% vs. 74%) among NPPV-treated patients compared with controls. This study included all patients with acute respiratory failure meeting entry criteria, not just COPD patients. When the COPD group was analyzed separately, the reduction in need for intubation among the NPPV-treated patients was even more dramatic, 9% versus 67%. Although morbidity and mortality rates, hospital lengths of stay, and hospital charges tended to decrease among the COPD patients, none of these were statistically significant, perhaps related to the small sample size.

The largest study,[14] a multicenter, randomized, prospective trial of NPPV using PSV via a face mask versus standard medical therapy alone in COPD patients also showed that the use of NPPV significantly reduced the need for endotracheal intubation (26% for NPPV vs. 74% for standard therapy, $p < 0.05$). In the subgroup successfully treated with NPPV, a significant improvement was noted in respiratory rate, as well as in PaO_2 at 1 hour and $PaCO_2$ at 12 hours. In addition, the frequency of complications (16% vs. 48%) and in-hospital mortality rate (9% vs. 29%) were significantly lower in the NPPV group compared with the conventional therapy group. Further, the length of hospital stay was significantly lower in the NPPV group (17 days vs. 35 days). The authors also found that regardless of which groups they were initially randomized to, patients who eventually required intubation had much higher morbidity and mortality rates than those who avoided intubation. The authors concluded that in *selected* patients with acute exacerbations of COPD, use of NPPV avoided the need for endotracheal intubation and its attendant complications, leading to reductions in morbidity and mortality rates. A more recent, smaller study by Celikel et al.[15] had similar conclusions, demonstrating a drastic reduction in the need for intubation (7% vs. 60%) and shorter lengths of hospital stay (10 days vs. 13 days) among NPPV-treated patients compared with controls.

In contrast to the above favorable studies, one small randomized trial (24 patients) concluded that NPPV was not useful in the therapy of acute COPD exacerbations.[16] However, this study encountered no intubations or mortality in either the NPPV group or controls, and the initial arterial blood gases indicated that patients were suffering milder exacerbations than was the case for patients entering the other randomized studies. Noninvasive ventilation cannot be shown to reduce intubations or mortality if none occur in the control group. Thus, a more satisfactory conclusion might have been that NPPV is not useful in COPD patients with mild exacerbations and should be reserved for patients with a greater need for ventilatory assistance.

Effects of NPPV on Duration of Ventilation and Length of Stay

Among the controlled trials, the duration of use of NPPV ranged from 4 hours to 20 hours per day for the first day, and rapidly fell during subsequent days. Kramer et al.,[13] observed an average use of 20 hours for the first 24-hour period, dropping to 14 hours for the second 24 hours, and only a few hours for the third, with an average duration of use of 3.3 days. Duration of use ranged from 1 to 9 hospital days, and a few patients continued to use NPPV after discharge to the home. Table 3 shows the length of ICU and hospital stays among NPPV patients compared with controls.

Although NPPV appeared to dramatically reduce the length of hospital stay in the Brochard study[14] and a small but statistically significant reduction was observed by Celikel et al.,[15] the finding was not consistent among all studies. It is also remarkable that there are such discrepancies in lengths of stay between the studies. For example, the average length of stay for controls in the Kramer study (17 days) is less than that for NPPV recipients in the Brochard study (22 days) despite quite similar blood gas and vital sign measures at the time of study entry. This suggests that factors besides medical considerations (i.e., reimbursement policies, bed availability, cultural practices with regard to hospitalization) may influence hospital bed utilization, and underlines the difficulty of comparing this variable between studies from different countries. It may be that NPPV reduces length of hospital stay in countries that tend to have long hospital stays, whereas it is difficult to demonstrate this benefit in countries that have aggressive hospital discharge policies.

Hospital Mortality

Table 4 shows the mortality of COPD patients with acute respiratory failure treated with NPPV compared with those treated conventionally among the controlled trials. Comparisons between studies are difficult because entry criteria, ventilator modes and settings, and medical treatment protocols differ. Only 2 studies showed a statistically

Table 4
Mortality Rate in Hospital

Reference	Patients (n)	Control %	NPPV %
Bott et al.[12]	60	30	10
Kramer et al.[13]	31	13	6
Brochard et al.[14]	85	29	9*
Vitacca et al.[18]	27	27	11*
Vitacca et al.[28]§	30	35	25*

Control patients underwent standard medical therapy in studies numbered 12–14, and invasive mechanical ventilation in study numbered 18. § Mortality in patients with pneumonia. *p < 0.05 for significant differences.

significant survival benefit,[12,14] and one of these[12] only after rejecting the intention-to-treat analysis. Nonetheless, throughout the studies, survival rates are consistently better for patients treated with NPPV than for those treated with medical therapy alone or with invasive mechanical ventilation.

Long-Term Survival

Some studies suggest that even a year after therapy, COPD patients treated acutely with NPPV instead of conventional therapy have reduced hospital stays and lower mortality rates, even when not placed on home mechanical ventilation after discharge (Table 5).[17-20] In a recent retrospective study,[20] COPD patients had mortality rates of 20% versus 26% in the ICU, 18% versus 48% at 3 months, and 29% versus 63% at 1 year, respectively, when treated with NPPV as opposed to invasive

Table 5
One Year Mortality after an Episode of Acute Respiratory Failure

Reference	No. of Patients	Treatment	Mortality
Nava[19]	42	Endotracheal intubation	45%
Confalonieri[20]	24	Standard medical	50%
Confalonieri[20]	24	NPPV	29%
Vitacca[18]*	27	Endotracheal intubation	63%
Vitacca[18]	30	NPPV	30%

*Mortality in patients with pneumonia.

positive pressure ventilation (IPPV). The number of repeat ICU admissions after discharge was also lower in NPPV patients. However, it is important to bear in mind that these studies were not randomized. In the absence of a clear explanation for why NPPV used in the acute situation would have such lasting benefits, it seems likely that these findings reflect a selection bias, with less ill patients undergoing NPPV during the acute exacerbations, and more severely ill ones (with a worse long-term prognosis) undergoing intubation.

Summary of Evidence

The evidence strongly supports the use of NPPV in patients with COPD exacerbations. The highest level of medical evidence is considered to be the randomized, controlled trial, and when multiple such trials support the use of a therapeutic intervention, that intervention is considered to have well-established benefits. However, the randomized trials supporting the use of NPPV for COPD exacerbations are not without limitations. Most have relatively small numbers, patient populations differ, and results are not entirely consistent between the studies. Nonetheless, when these studies were subjected to a meta-analysis, the reductions in the need for intubation and mortality rates proved to be highly statistically significant.[21] In addition, the studies show that clinicians can expect prompt improvements in respiratory rates, gas exchange, and sensation of respiratory distress when patients with acute COPD exacerbations are treated with NPPV. Reductions in complication rates and in-hospital lengths of stay proved harder to assess because of inconsistencies between the studies. Despite the limitations, however, NPPV should now be considered the ventilator modality of first choice for *selected* patients with COPD exacerbations. The word selected is emphasized because careful patient selection is key to the safe and successful application of NPPV, and this process will be discussed in detail in the following section.

Selection of Patients with COPD Exacerbations to Receive NPPV

Determinants of Success

Although results with NPPV have been promising, failure rates have consistently been observed in approximately 10–40% of patients.

When NPPV fails, its use might be viewed as delaying endotracheal intubation, with possible increased risk to the patient.[22] Accordingly, the prompt identification of those most apt to succeed or fail becomes important. Several studies have identified predictors of success or failure, and these are listed in Table 6.[23,24]

These studies indicate that patients with at least some hypercapnia are more likely to succeed than those without, but that excessive hypercapnia (and acidemia) lower the likelihood of success. Likewise, Acute Physiology Assessment Chronic Health Evaluation II (APACHE II) scores are elevated, as would be expected in these acutely ill patients, but very high APACHE II scores predict failure. Some of the factors that predict success are obvious, such as the ability to cooperate (or better neurologic scores), manageable secretions, and less air leak through the mouth in patients receiving nasal ventilation. Patients with pneumonia (presumably because of increased secretions) and edentulous patients (because of increased air leak) have been reported to have worse outcomes in some studies.[23,24] Of note, numerous reports have found that a reduction in respiratory and heart rates, good synchrony with the ventilator, and improvement in $PaCO_2$ within the first 2 hours are highly predictive of success. Therefore, the initial severity of the episode of acute respiratory failure and the level of acidosis and hypercapnia after a brief trial of NPPV allow the clinician to make a judgment about continuing treatment.[24]

Selection Criteria

Based on criteria used in the randomized, controlled trials,[12-16] an algorithm for the selection of patients with COPD exacerbations to

---

Table 6
Determinants of Success vs. Failure for NPPV[12,14,19–21]

Better neurological status
Cooperative
Less acidosis and hypercapnia on admission
Lesser severity of illness as indicated by APACHE II score
Intact dentition
Less air leaking
No pneumonia
Controllable secretions
Improved vital signs, pH and $PaCO_2$ within 2 hours of initiation

---

receive NPPV is presented in Table 7. The selection process can be seen as a simple 2-step process. The first step is to identify patients who are sufficiently ill to warrant ventilatory assistance and to screen out those who are apt to recover uneventfully without it. Patients should have clinical and physiologic evidence of acute ventilatory failure, including acute respiratory acidosis, tachypnea, use of accessory muscles of inspiration, or abdominal paradox. Alternatively, COPD patients with mainly acute hypoxemic respiratory failure may be considered candidates, although controlled studies to support this indication are lacking, and available evidence suggests that success rates are lower in the absence of any CO_2 retention.[25]

The second step is to exclude patients who have contraindications because they are too ill to be safely managed noninvasively or they are too likely to fail (Table 8). For example, patients with respiratory arrest or hypotensive shock are too ill, and uncooperative patients are too likely to fail to permit use of NPPV.[10] Finally, at least partial reversal of the exacerbation should be anticipated within hours or days. COPD patients with superimposed severe medical instability of copious secretions are best managed invasively.

Table 7
Suggested Algorithm for Ventilatory Management of Acute
Exacerbations of COPD

Screening
 STEP 1. Patient has evidence of acute decompensation: *ph < 7.35, PaCO₂ > 45, RR > 25, increased respiratory distress (abdominal paradox, accessory muscle use, etc)*.
  IF NO: Conventional treatment.
  IF YES: Go to Step 2.
 STEP 2. Patient has contraindication to NPPV (see Table 8).
  IF YES: Consider endotracheal intubation.
  IF NO: NPPV.
Adaptation
 Patient is on NPPV; check vital signs, blood gases, synchrony with ventilator after 1–2 hours.
  IF IMPROVED: Continue on NPPV and attempt weaning.
  IF NOT: Endotracheal intubation.
  IF endotracheal intubation is necessary: Consider early extubation and NPPV to facilitate weaning.

Table 8
Contraindications to Mask Ventilation

Respiratory arrest
Uncooperative patient
Medically unstable patient, e.g:
  Hemodynamically unstable
  Severe gastrointestinal bleeding
Inability to protect airway
Excessive airway secretions
Impaired cough or swallowing mechanism

Because they screen out patients who are too mildly or severely ill to receive noninvasive ventilation, the appropriate application of these guidelines identifies only a minority, albeit a substantial minority, of patients with COPD exacerbations who prove to be good candidates for NPPV. In the controlled study of Brochard et al.,[14] only 31% of patients with COPD who were hospitalized during the study period met the criteria for enrollment.

Application of NPPV to COPD Patients

The practical application of NPPV to patients has been discussed in detail in prior chapters. Considerations pertinent to COPD patients will be discussed here.

Location

Studies on the use of NPPV in acute COPD exacerbations have initiated ventilation in an emergency room,[13] ICU, or respiratory intermediate care unit (RICU),[13,14] or on a general ward.[12,20] Ideally, the choice of location should depend on the patient's need for monitoring as determined by the level of acuity. Patients who are at high risk of deterioration in the event of discontinuation require close monitoring, but as they stabilize, transfer to less intensive settings such as general medical wards may be appropriate. NPPV offers the possibility of more efficient utilization of care in this regard, because it can be easily implemented in RICUs at less cost than in ICUs, and it permits expedited transfers off these units if the weaning process is facilitated.[26]

Interface Selection

Some practitioners argue that COPD patients are "mouth breathers," particularly during bouts of acute respiratory distress and should be treated routinely with oronasal masks. Others argue that many of these patients are accustomed to nasal oxygen, have a low tolerance level for bulky facial devices, and should be treated initially with nasal masks. The truth is that there are no convincing data one way or the other, and uncontrolled studies in the literature suggest that success rates are similar regardless of the mask type used. However, proper fitting is of paramount importance. For this reason, the practitioner should keep a variety of mask types and sizes in a "mask bag" attached to a noninvasive ventilator cart. The use of "fitting gauges" provided by mask manufacturers is also encouraged.

Selection of a Ventilator

The issues relating to selection of a "critical care" versus a "bilevel" type of ventilator are discussed in Chapter 1. No studies have directly compared the various types, but success rates appear to be comparable. A comparative study has shown that triggering capabilities of most bilevel ventilators are as good as, or significantly better than, critical care ventilators.[27] Further, patients with COPD exacerbations usually have mild to moderate oxygenation defects and do not require the oxygen blending capability of a critical care ventilator. Therefore, either type of ventilator could be selected with equal expectations of success.

Selection of a Ventilator Mode

Pressure support ventilation and volume-limited modes have both been used to successfully deliver NPPV to COPD patients. In controlled studies, both modes have shown similar effectiveness in improving arterial blood gases and avoiding endotracheal intubation. In a recent physiologic study, volume-limited ventilation was slightly more effective at providing respiratory muscle rest, but subjective respiratory discomfort was less with PSV.[27] Also, in an earlier study, patient compliance was rated better with PSV than with volume-limited ventilation.[28] Thus, PSV is currently considered preferable to volume-limited A/C ventilation. However, it should be borne in mind that because of the short inspiratory duration and high inspiratory flow rate used by some patients during COPD exacerbations, flow-cycled modes like PSV may have difficulty sensing the onset of patient expiration. Patients may have to exert considerable expiratory force to cycle the ventilator, adding to the work of breathing and, potentially, to patient discomfort.[29] Based on preliminary evidence,[30] modes such as proportional assist ventilation that are not prone to this problem may prove to be even more comfortable than PSV.

Ventilator Settings

Initial settings, of course, depend on the ventilator mode selected. With pressure-limited modes, initial total inspiratory positive airway pressure (IPAP) has been 10–12 mm H_2O in most studies, but pressures have ranged from 8–20 cm H_2O. For volume-limited modes, tidal volumes of 10–15 mL/kg are most often used. In adjusting initial inspiratory pressures or volumes, the aim should be to provide enough assistance to unload the respiratory muscles without causing excessive patient discomfort. It should be recalled that partial assistance is usually sufficient, and that excessive pressures may render patients intolerant.

Expiratory pressure (usually 4–6 cm H_2O) should also be applied to counterbalance auto-PEEP and to provide sufficient bias flow to minimize rebreathing.[31] PEEPe can be adjusted upward after initiation to facilitate triggering in patients with suspected auto-PEEP, or to improve oxygenation in patients with acute hypoxemic respiratory failure. The difference between the total inspiratory pressure and PEEP is the level of pressure support, so high levels of PEEP will necessitate high inspiratory pressures if the support level is to be maintained. Some pressure-limited ventilators permit adjustment of "rise time," inspiratory duration, or cycling sensitivity. Considering that some COPD patients prefer high inspiratory flow rates[32] and that PSV modes may have problems sensing the onset of expiration,[29] these may be useful in optimizing patient-ventilator synchrony, and hence, comfort.

With both pressure- and volume-limited modes, a backup rate is usually provided, partly to assure continued ventilation in the event of apneas, and also to make certain that the ventilator cycles in the presence of air leaks that inevitably occur during NPPV. Ventilators may have difficulty sensing patient breathing efforts in the presence of leaks, so a backup rate slightly below the patient's spontaneous breathing rate will sustain the ventilator triggering rate even in the presence of leaks.

Oxygenation, Humidification, and Other Considerations

For critical care ventilators, O_2 can be provided via the blender, just as for invasive ventilation. For portable bilevel ventilators, O_2 is provided via a port in the mask or into the ventilator circuitry via a "T" connector. In either case, desired O_2 saturation targets (usually >90–92%) are generally easily met by simple titration. Because they are receiving ventilatory assistance, severe CO_2 retainers usually tolerate O_2 supplementation without greater CO_2 retention, unlike the situation with unassisted breathing.

Because physiologic upper airway air conditioning mechanisms are left intact during NPPV, humidification is not necessary for acute applications. However, some patients complain of drying related to air leaks, so passover-type humidifiers can be used. Humidification may also be indicated for COPD patients with copious thick secretions. Heated passover-type humidifiers are more efficient than nonheated ones. Heat and moisture exchangers should be avoided because these may increase resistance in the tubing and tend to accumulate secretions that could be problematic in COPD patients. Along these lines, aerosolized bronchodilator treatments can be administered via the ventilator[33] or by temporary interruption of therapy. For acutely ill patients who may not tolerate temporary cessation of therapy, administration via the ventilator is preferred.

Role of Nurses and Therapists

The success of noninvasive ventilation depends on close staff supervision by nurses, physiotherapists, and/or respiratory therapists (Table 9). In the United States, respiratory therapists are usually responsible for initiating NPPV once the physician has decided that it is indicated.

Table 9
Staff Responsibilities for Initiation of NPPV

- Select appropriate patient.
- Optimize mask type and fit.
- Choose appropriate ventilator.
- Optimize ventilator settings.
- Select appropriate location.
- Monitor patient according to acuity of illness.
- Check periodically on patient's tolerance and acceptance.
- Oversee weaning or continue NPPV if deemed necessary.

In Europe, nurses may be responsible for initiating NPPV and, on either continent, they are critical in helping patients to adapt and continue therapy. Experienced clinicians must be present at the bedside to properly fit the interface and adjust the ventilator, impart a sense of confidence about the likelihood of success, and encourage the patient to relax and breathe in synchrony with the ventilator. One study has shown that a broad educational program for physicians, therapists, and nurses is essential for successful implementation of NPPV.[34]

Chevrolet et al.[35] raised concerns about the expenditure of nursing time required to administer NPPV to patients with obstructive diseases, but others have found that nurses encountered no more difficulty[12] and required no more time[13] to treat COPD patients with mask ventilation than for standard therapy. In one study,[13] respiratory therapists tended to spend more time during the initial shift at the bedside of patients receiving NPPV compared with control patients, but this time expenditure fell significantly by the second shift. Nava et al.[34] have recently shown that in an experienced RICU, NPPV is neither more time consuming nor more costly to provide than endotracheal intubation. Regardless of whether time consumption is greater or less than invasive ventilation, patients receiving NPPV require periodic checks to assure that they are using it optimally, and to assist with weaning.

Weaning COPD Patients from Mechanical Ventilation

The most often used approach to weaning NPPV from COPD patients resembles T-piece weaning.[12,13] Patients recovering from a COPD exacerbation are usually ready to initiate weaning trials within 1–3 days of initiation, and the average patient will wean within 2–3 days. Some patients have difficulty weaning and must use NPPV most of the time for extended periods of time. Problems may arise from mask intolerance or nasal ulcers, and this practice may raise ethical concerns in patients who have stated that they wish no life support. However, as long as the patient understands that NPPV is being used for life support in this circumstance and wishes to continue, our practice is to continue as long as the patient desires. A minority of COPD patients treated with NPPV for an acute exacerbation will continue nocturnal ventilatory support.

The Health Care Financing Agency (HCFA) in the United States has recently published guidelines for the use of long-term NPPV in patients with COPD (see Chapter 11 for details). In addition to hypercapnia ($PaCO_2$ >52 mm Hg), these patients must have O_2 desaturations of < 88% for at least 5 consecutive minutes while using O_2 at their usual flow rate, and obstructive sleep apnea must be excluded. Presently, these patients must also undergo an initial trial of 2 months using assisted ventilation without a backup rate, although this guideline may be modified. The HCFA guidelines notwithstanding, patients with frequent hospitalizations due to exacerbations of COPD may be good candidates for long-term NPPV because of possible reductions in hospital use.

Another possible use of NPPV in patients recovering from bouts of acute respiratory failure due to COPD is as a technique to facilitate weaning from invasive ventilation. This is discussed in detail in Chapter 6.

Conclusions

NPPV represents an advance in the therapy of patents with acute respiratory failure due to COPD and is currently considered the ventilatory modality of first choice in appropriately selected patients. Patients should be selected using standard guidelines, aimed at excluding patients who are too mildly ill to be aided by ventilatory assistance, and those who are too ill and would be at higher risk if managed noninvasively. NPPV should be administered by an experienced staff, with attention paid to proper fitting of the mask, adjustment of the ventilator, and optimizing comfort for the patient. When treating COPD patients with NPPV according to these general management guidelines, practitioners must be sensitive to the problems that are characteristic of this patient population, including auto-PEEP and patient-ventilator asynchrony caused by failure to promptly cycle. Adding PEEPe or adjusting inspiratory termination criteria may be very helpful in enhancing patient-ventilator synchrony and overall comfort. When administered to properly selected COPD patients by a skilled staff, we can expect reductions in the use of invasive ventilation, lower complication and mortality rates, shorter hospital stays and, ultimately, reduced health care costs.

References

1. Muir JF, Similowski T, Derenne JP. Oxygen therapy during acute respiratory failure of chronic obstructive pulmonary disease. In Derenne JP, Whitelaw WA, Similowski T (eds). Acute Respiratory Failure in Chronic Obstructive Pulmonary Disease. New York, Marcel Dekker, 1996, pp 579-588.

2. Tobin MJ. Mechanical ventilation. N Engl J Med 1994;130:1056-1061.
3. Pingleton SK, Rossi A. Respiratory and non respiratory complications of critical illness. In Parrillo JE, Bone RC (eds). Critical Care Medicine: Principles of Diagnosis and Management. St. Louis, Mosby, 1995, pp 755-780.
4. Carrey Z, Gottfried S, Levy R. Ventilatory muscle support in respiratory failure with nasal positive-pressure ventilation. Chest 1990;97:150-158.
5. Nava S, Ambrosino N, Rubini F, et al. Effect of nasal pressure support ventilation and external PEEP on diaphragmatic activity in patients with severe stable COPD. Chest 1993;103:143-150.
6. Appendini L, Patessio A, Zanaboni S, et al. Physiological effects of positive end expiratory pressure and mask pressure support during exacerbations of chronic obstructive pulmonary disease. Am J Respir Crit Care Med 1994;149:1069-1076.
7. Meyer TJ, Hill NS. Noninvasive positive pressure ventilation to treat respiratory failure. Ann Intern Med 1994;120:760-770.
8. Sassoon CSH. Noninvasive positive-pressure ventilation in acute respiratory failure: review of reported experience with special attention to use during weaning. Respir Care 1995;40:282-288.
9. Meduri GU. Noninvasive positive-pressure ventilation in patients with acute respiratory failure. Clin Chest Med 1996;17:513-552.
10. Ambrosino N. Noninvasive mechanical ventilation in acute respiratory failure. Eur Respir J 1996;9:795-807.
11. Hillberg RE, Johnson DC. Noninvasive ventilation. N Engl J Med 1997; 337:1746-1752.
12. Bott J, Carroll MP, Conway JH, et al. Randomized controlled trial of nasal ventilation in acute ventilatory failure due to chronic obstructive airways disease. Lancet 1993;341:1555-1557.
13. Kramer N, Meyer TJ, Meharg J, et al. Randomized, prospective trial of noninvasive positive pressure ventilation in acute respiratory failure. Am J Respir Crit Care Med 1995;151:1799-1806.
14. Brochard L, Mancebo J, Wysocki M, et al. Noninvasive ventilation for acute exacerbations of chronic obstructive pulmonary disease. N Engl J Med 1995;333:817-822.
15. Celikel T, Sungur M, Ceyhan B, Karakurt S. Comparison of noninvasive positive pressure ventilation with standard medical therapy in hypercapnic acute respiratory failure. Chest 1998;114:1636-1642.
16. Barbe F, Quera-Salva MA, de Lattre J, et al. Long-term effects of nasal intermittent positive pressure ventilation on pulmonary function and sleep architecture in patients with neuromuscular diseases. Chest 1996; 110:1179-1183.
17. Connors AF, Dawson NV, Thomas C, et al. Outcomes following acute exacerbation of severe chronic obstructive lung disease. Am J Respir Crit Care Med 1996;154:959-967.
18. Vitacca M, Clini E, Rubini F, et al. Noninvasive mechanical ventilation in severe COPD and acute respiratory failure: short and long term prognosis. Intensive Care Med 1996;22:94-100.
19. Nava S, Rubini F, Zanotti E, et al. Survival and prediction of successful ventilator weaning in COPD patients requiring mechanical ventilation for more than 21 days. Eur Respir J 1994;7:1645-1652.

20. Confalonieri M, Parigi P, Scartabellati A, et al. Noninvasive mechanical ventilation improves the immediate and long-term outcome of COPD patients with acute respiratory failure. Eur Respir J 1996;9:422-430.
21. Keenan SP, Kernerman PD, Cook DJ, et al. The effect of noninvasive positive pressure ventilation on mortality in patients admitted with acute respiratory failure: a meta-analysis. Crit Care Med 1997;25:1685-1692.
22. Wood KA, Lewis L, Von Harz B, Kollef MH. The use of noninvasive positive pressure ventilation in the emergency department. Chest 1998; 113:1339-1346.
23. Ambrosino N, Foglio K, Rubini F, et al. Noninvasive mechanical ventilation in acute respiratory failure due to chronic obstructive pulmonary disease: correlates for success. Thorax 1995;50:755-757.
24. Soo Hoo GW, Santiago S, Williams A. Nasal mechanical ventilation for hypercapnic respiratory failure in chronic obstructive pulmonary disease: determinants of success and failure. Crit Care Med 1994;22:1253-1261.
25. Wysocki M, Laurent T, Wolff MA, et al. Noninvasive pressure support ventilation in patients with acute respiratory failure: a randomized comparison with conventional therapy. Chest 1995;107:761-768.
26. Nava S, Ambrosino N, Clini E, et al. Noninvasive mechanical ventilation in the weaning of patients with respiratory failure due to chronic obstructive pulmonary disease: a randomized study. Ann Intern Med 1998;128:721-728.
27. Girault C, Richard JC, Chevron V, et al. Comparative physiologic effects of noninvasive assist-control and pressure support ventilation in acute hypercapnic respiratory failure. Chest 1997;111:1639-1648.
28. Vitacca M, Rubini F, Foglio K, et al. Noninvasive modalities of positive pressure ventilation improve the outcome of acute exacerbations in COPD patients. Intensive Care Med 1993;9:450-455.
29. Jubran A, Van de Graffe WB, Tobin MJ. Variability of patient-ventilator interaction with pressure support ventilation in patients with chronic obstructive pulmonary disease. Am J Respir Crit Care Med 1995;152:129-136.
30. Gay P, Heil D, Hollets S, et al. A randomized, prospective trial of noninvasive proportional assist ventilation (PAV) to treat acute respiratory insufficiency (ARI). Am J Respir Crit Care Med 1999;159:A14.
31. Lofaso F, Brochard L, Hang T, et al. Home versus intensive care pressure support devices: experimental and clinical comparison. Am J Respir Crit Care Med 1996;153:1591-1599.
32. Bonmarchand G, Chevron V, Chopin C, et al. Increased initial flow rate reduces inspiratory work of breathing during pressure support ventilation in patients with exacerbation of chronic obstructive pulmonary disease. Intensive Care Med 1996;22:1147-1154.
33. Pollack C Jr, Torres MT, Alexander L. Feasibility study of the use of bilevel positive airway pressure for respiratory support in the emergency department. Ann Emerg Med 1996; 27:189-192.
34. Nava S, Evangelisti I, Rampulla C, et al. Human and financial costs of noninvasive mechanical ventilation in patients affected by COPD and acute respiratory failure. Chest 1997;111:1631-1638.
35. Chevrolet JC, Jolliet P, Abajo B, et al. Nasal positive pressure ventilation in patients with acute respiratory failure. Chest 1991;100:445-454.

Chapter 5

Noninvasive Positive Pressure Ventilation for Non Chronic Obstructive Pulmonary Disease Causes of Acute Respiratory Failure

Nicholas S. Hill, M.D.

Introduction

The best established indication for noninvasive positive pressure ventilation (NPPV) in the acute setting is for chronic obstructive pulmonary disease (COPD) exacerbations, as discussed in Chapter 4. However, there are numerous other etiologies of acute respiratory failure for which application of NPPV may be appropriate. For most of these, the level of evidence is not as strong as it is for COPD, but some evidence is usually available. The following summarizes the evidence supporting use of NPPV for non-COPD etiologies and makes recommendations for patient selection and NPPV implementation. As a general rule, the principles outlined for selecting patients with acute respiratory insufficiency due to COPD exacerbations to receive NPPV can be applied to other forms of acute respiratory failure, but with modifications depending on the disease process. In addition, although it is not technically a form of ventilatory assistance because it does not actively assist inspiration, continuous positive airway pressure (CPAP) alone has potential as a respiratory aid for some forms of respiratory failure, and its appropriate application will be discussed.

Specific Etiologies of Respiratory Failure

Non-COPD Obstructive Diseases

Asthma

The success of NPPV in treating acute exacerbations of COPD has led many clinicians to surmise that it should be effective in acute

From *Noninvasive Positive Pressure Ventilation: Principles and Applications,* edited by Nicholas S. Hill. © 2001, Futura Publishing Company, Inc., Armonk, NY.

exacerbations due to other obstructive etiologies, as well. Accordingly, several reports have appeared on the use of NPPV for acute asthma exacerbations.[1-4] Most reports consist of series of patients with a variety of respiratory disorders and have included 2 or fewer asthma patients.[1,2] However, Meduri et al.[3] included 5 patients with acute asthma in their study of 158 patients with acute respiratory failure treated with face mask NPPV. The average initial $PaCO_2$ among these asthma patients was 67 mm Hg, only 1 required intubation, and there were no mortalities. In a subsequent study,[4] the same authors applied face mask pressure support ventilation (PSV) (14 ± 5 cm H_2O) with positive end-expiratory pressure (PEEP) (4 ± 2 cm H_2O) to 17 asthma patients with an average initial pH of 7.25 and $PaCO_2$ of 65 mm Hg. Dyspnea was rapidly relieved, only 2 patients required intubation (for increasing $PaCO_2$), the average duration of ventilation was 16 hours, and no complications occurred. The authors concluded that NPPV appears to be highly effective in correcting gas exchange abnormalities and avoiding intubation in patients with acute severe asthma. However, the lack of controls and the absence of well-defined selection criteria in these studies weaken the conclusions.

Selection of patients with acute asthma to receive NPPV is complicated by the tendency of this disease to change rapidly over time, and much more than for COPD. Some patients come to an emergency department with extreme dyspnea but respond rapidly to bronchodilators and would not likely benefit from NPPV. Others come to the emergency department in a moribund state and require prompt intubation. Those most likely to benefit from NPPV fall between these extremes, but in the absence of controlled trials, specific selection criteria have not been confirmed and the following recommendations on patient selection are tentative.

As listed in Table 1, patients with moderate to severe dyspnea who have not responded promptly to aerosolized bronchodilator treatments are appropriate candidates. Because severe exacerbations of asthma, in contrast to those of COPD, are characterized by marked increases in inspiratory as well as expiratory resistance, respiratory rates tend to be higher. Accordingly, a respiratory rate of ≥ 28 breaths/min is suggested as a threshold value for asthmatics as opposed to the 24 breaths/min suggested for COPD, with accessory muscle use or abdominal paradox retained as indicators of excessive respiratory muscle work. In addition, a $PaCO_2$ value of > 40 mm Hg is suggested as a threshold value for asthmatics, considering that chronic CO_2 retention is not a feature of the disease and a normal $PaCO_2$ value will occur during the "crossover" from hyperventilation to hypoventilation.[5,6] In general, the

Table 1
Suggested Selection and Exclusion
Guidelines for use of NPPV in Acute Asthma

Selection
Clinical
  Moderate to severe respiratory distress
  Tachypnea (RR > 28 breaths/min)
  Accessory muscle use or paradoxical breathing and no prompt response to
    bronchodilators
Gas Exchange
  $PaCO_2$ > 40 mmHg or rising $PaCO_2$
  PaO_2/FiO_2 < 200

Exclusion
  Respiratory arrest
  Moribund or comatose
  pH < 7.10
  Medically unstable; systolic BP < 90 mmHg
  Uncooperative
  Excessive secretions
  Unable to protect airway
  Unable to fit mask

RR, respiratory rate; BP, blood pressure.

clinical assessment that a patient is at risk for developing respiratory muscle fatigue can be used as an indication for NPPV, and outweighs any blood gas criteria proposed. However, some patients are probably too ill to be managed safely with NPPV, such as those with severe CO_2 retention and acidemia, and intubation should not be delayed in these patients by a misguided NPPV trial.

The decision to initiate NPPV for a patient with acute asthma is also complicated by the availability of a number of alternative therapies. For example, magnesium[7] or heliox[8] may be used as rescue therapies at many emergency departments, and it has not been determined whether NPPV should be reserved for patients who fail these, or whether it should be used in combination with heliox. Considering that NPPV has also been used as a way to administer aerosolized bronchodilator therapy,[9] one approach to the severe acute asthmatic would be to provide NPPV promptly upon admission to an emergency room. NPPV would thus serve as a vehicle for administration of bronchodilators while providing some ventilatory assistance, much as intermittent positive pressure breathing (IPPB) was used in the past.[10] Until more studies are available to guide clinical decision making, the choices between these options will be left largely up to individual clinician judgment.

Cystic Fibrosis

Cystic fibrosis shares many pathophysiologic features with COPD, including severe expiratory airway obstruction and the propensity to develop dynamic hyperinflation and auto-PEEP during acute exacerbations. In addition, the worsening in airway obstruction during exacerbations may be small, but enough to precipitate respiratory muscle fatigue, as occurs in COPD patients. Therefore, use of NPPV as a means of partial ventilatory support in cystic fibrosis patients would be expected to provide benefit similar to that seen in COPD patients. Although this has not been proven in controlled trials, case series suggest that NPPV can be used successfully for this indication. Hodson et al.[11] described the use of NPPV to treat end-stage cystic fibrosis patients with forced expiratory volume in 1 second (FEV_1) ranging from 350 mL to 800 mL and with severe acute-on-chronic CO_2 retention (initial $PaCO_2$ ranging from 63 mm Hg to 112 mm Hg). All 6 patients had initial improvement or at least stabilization of gas exchange and were supported for periods ranging from 3 days to 36 days with NPPV. Four of the patients survived until a heart-lung transplantation could be performed. This study illustrates the potential utility of NPPV as a rescue therapy in supporting acutely deteriorating cystic fibrosis patients and in providing a "bridge to transplantation."[11]

As is the case with most non-COPD causes of acute respiratory failure, the lack of controlled trials precludes the provision of firm selection criteria for patients with cystic fibrosis to receive NPPV. On the other hand, considering that cystic fibrosis is a form of chronic airway obstruction that shares many pathophysiologic features with COPD, the same selection criteria may be applied (see the selection algorithm provided in Chapter 4, Table 7). Because thickened secretions are more often seen with cystic fibrosis than with COPD, clinicians should consider use of a nasal, rather than an oronasal, mask to facilitate expectoration, and they should be prepared to administer aerosolized medications via the NPPV ventilator circuit.

Obstructive Sleep Apnea

Severe obstructive sleep apnea can cause CO_2 retention and cor pulmonale. If left untreated, this condition can intensify so that patients present to acute care hospitals with acute-on-chronic respiratory failure in a pre-terminal state. Sturani et al.[12] described the successful use of nasal NPPV administered using a BiPAP™ (Respironics, Inc., Murrysville, PA) device to 5 such patients presenting with confusion or obtundation and an average initial $PaCO_2$ of 77 mm Hg. After 1 to 3 hours, average $PaCO_2$ fell to 63 mm Hg, and endotracheal intubation was avoided in all cases. Piper and Sullivan[13] described 13 similar patients with morbid obesity (body mass index >35) and severe CO_2 retention (average $PaCO_2$, 62 mm Hg) who were subacutely ill and responded favorably to the institution of NPPV. Most were able to switch to CPAP after several weeks of NPPV therapy.

Severe obstructive sleep apnea patients are often morbidly obese and require unusually high inspiratory pressures to assist ventilation because of the high respiratory impedance posed by the chest wall. In such situations, use of a volume-limited ventilator may be successful to achieve the high inspiratory pressures necessary (35–40 cm H_2O) when pressure-limited ventilation using bilevel ventilators has been unsuccessful.[13] The positive pressure not only helps to overcome respiratory impedance due to the large chest wall mass, but also helps to "stent" the upper airway, preventing inspiratory collapse of upper airway structures. Further, these patients characteristically have blunting of central respiratory drive, and assisted ventilation with reversal of severe CO_2 retention usually helps to restore, at least partially, central sensitivity to CO_2.

Selection of patients with acute respiratory failure due to advanced obstructive sleep apnea has not previously been discussed in the literature. It should be based on the patient's need for ventilatory assistance as determined by the severity of respiratory distress (which may be minimal if CO_2 accumulation has been gradual), severity of CO_2 retention and acidosis, and lack of contraindications for NPPV that would dictate the need for intubation. The choice between CPAP and NPPV (with active inspiratory assistance) is also a matter of clinical judgment in such patients, but those with moderate to severe CO_2 retention and acidemia ($PaCO_2$ >50 mm Hg, pH <7.30) would seem to be better candidates for NPPV.

Upper Airway Obstruction

Use of NPPV to support patients with acute respiratory failure due to upper airway obstruction has been reported in only small case series. Of the 158 patients in the series of Meduri et al.,[3] 3 had upper airway obstruction, 2 of whom avoided intubation. As a temporizing measure to avoid intubation, NPPV would seem to be a sensible approach. In addition to providing assistance for fatiguing inspiratory muscles, NPPV also provides positive pressure to the upper airway, which could help to widen the airway, prevent phasic narrowing, and reduce resistance if there is any reversible component to the obstruction.

No selection criteria have been proposed for application of NPPV to patients with acute upper airway obstruction, but those used for COPD patients would seem to be applicable. Patients in moderate to severe respiratory distress who have manifestations of impending respiratory muscle fatigue, including accessory muscle use or abdominal paradox, or those with any CO_2 retention, should be considered for NPPV therapy. In addition, a combination of NPPV with heliox should be considered as a way to further decrease upper airway resistance. Judgment must be exercised in excluding patients who are poor candidates for NPPV. Obviously, if upper airway obstruction is complete (as may occur with acute epiglottitis, for instance) intubation should not be delayed.

Restrictive Diseases

Restrictive Thoracic Diseases

One of the best-accepted applications of NPPV is to provide ventilatory assistance to patients with chronic respiratory failure due to restrictive thoracic diseases. However, use of NPPV to treat acute respiratory failure in patients with thoracic restriction has received relatively little attention, perhaps because they comprise only a small proportion of patients presenting to acute care hospitals with acute respiratory failure. In the Meduri et al. large study that enrolled all eligible patients admitted to an intensive care unit over a 2-year period, only 5 of 158 patients had restrictive diseases.[3] On the other hand, some anecdotal case series report that NPPV alleviates gas exchange abnormalities and avoids intubation in neuromuscular disease[14] and kyphoscoliotic[15] patients with acute respiratory failure.

Bach et al.[16] described a regimen for managing acute deteriorations in patients with chronic respiratory failure due to neuromuscular disease. These patients were already using noninvasive ventilation at home, and increased the duration of use to 24 hours per day during exacerbations while pulse oximetry was continuously monitored. If

O_2 saturation fell below 90%, aggressive removal of secretions was undertaken using manually assisted coughing and mechanical aids such as the cough In-Exsufflator (JH Emerson, Cambridge, MA)[17] (see Chapter 1) until oxygen saturation returned to above 90%. Although no controlled studies have established the efficacy of this approach, its use during acute exacerbations appears to permit patients to remain at home, with a dramatic reduction in the need for hospitalization.

When an aggressive approach such as that outlined above is implemented to keep patients at home during acute exacerbations, the need for hospitalization usually means that secretion retention has become an overwhelming problem. Further efforts to support patients noninvasively will often be futile. Excessive delays before intubation should be avoided, because management may sometimes be facilitated by temporary intubation to clear retained secretions, followed by extubation and resumption of NPPV once the situation has stabilized.

For success, the approach described by Bach et al. requires highly trained and committed caregivers in the home. For patients lacking these resources, earlier hospitalization will be necessary. To continue NPPV and avoid intubation in these patients, the hospital staff must be sensitized to the special needs of this patient population. The patients often have special positioning needs, and because they are seen relatively infrequently in general hospital units compared with other causes of respiratory deterioration, nursing and respiratory therapy staff often need re-education in the proper application of cough assistive techniques.[18] Without these, the likelihood of success with NPPV is much lower once these patients have been hospitalized.

Restrictive Lung Diseases

No information is available on NPPV therapy for patients with acutely deteriorating restrictive lung diseases such as interstitial fibrosis. Theoretically, such patients would be difficult to manage noninvasively, because of the severe reductions in lung compliance and the need for high inflation pressures that are likely to be poorly tolerated. Further, this application would not be recommended unless an acute reversible superimposed condition was thought to be responsible for the deterioration.

Acute Respiratory Failure Without Prior Lung Disease

This category refers to patients who have no underlying chronic lung condition and, therefore, present with entirely acute (or "de novo"[19]) as opposed to acute-on-chronic respiratory failure. In this case, stabilization may require a more complete reversal of the respiratory deterioration than is the case with acute-on-chronic respiratory failure, where reversal of a relatively small acute component may be adequate to restore stability. Perhaps for this reason, some reports suggest that NPPV is less successful in patients without prior chronic lung disease,[20] although this has not been proven. Nonetheless, clinicians should be particularly cautious about selection criteria in this group of patients, avoiding those with severe respiratory deteriorations that are unlikely to be reversed within days.

Adult Respiratory Distress Syndrome

The use of NPPV in the adult respiratory distress syndrome (ARDS) has been reported in a few case series. Meduri et al.[1] administered NPPV to 3 ARDS patients in their series, 2 of whom required intubation. More recently, Rocker et al.[21] described the use of NPPV in 10 patients with 12 episodes of ARDS; 6 of these patients eventually required intubation. NPPV was successful in two-thirds of the patients when it was used as the initial mode of mechanical ventilation. These studies show that NPPV can be used to successfully support patients with ARDS, but no controlled trials have been performed to demonstrate improvements in outcome variables besides avoidance of intubation. Further, selection criteria have not been discussed in the case series.

Considering the dearth of clinical information, the severity of the gas exchange defects, and the prolonged duration of respiratory failure in many patients with ARDS, application of NPPV is not recommended for most of these patients. A trial of NPPV could be attempted in those with moderate to severe respiratory distress, a high likelihood of early reversal, and no instability of other organ systems, but without very severe gas exchange defects (e.g., $PaO_2/FiO_2 >100$) (Table 2). However, they should be closely observed and promptly intubated if they continue to deteriorate, so that inordinate delays in needed interventions are avoided.

Cardiogenic Pulmonary Edema

Application of CPAP to patients with acute pulmonary edema was first described during the 1930s.[22] Although not a true ventilatory mode because it does not actively assist inspiration, CPAP has been used for

Table 2
Suggested Selection and Exclusion
Guidelines for Use of NPPV in Patients with ARDS

Selection
Clinical
   Moderate to severe dyspnea
   Accessory muscle use or abdominal paradox
   Tachypnea: RR > 30–35 breaths/min
   Perceived likelihood of early reversal
Gas Exchange
   $PaO_2/FiO_2 < 200$

Exclusion
   Very severe respiratory distress or apnea
   Medically unstable, systolic BP < 90 mm Hg despite pressors; severe sepsis
   Likelihood of prolonged respiratory failure, multiorgan system failure
   $PaO_2/FiO_2 < 100$
   Agitated or uncooperative
   Comatose
   Unable to protect airway or fit mask
   Excessive secretions

various forms of acute respiratory failure. By delivering a constant pressure during both inspiration and expiration, CPAP increases functional residual capacity and opens collapsed or underventilated alveoli, thus decreasing right-to-left intrapulmonary shunt and improving oxygenation. The opening of alveoli and increase in functional residual capacity may also improve lung compliance, decreasing the work of breathing.[23] In addition, by lowering ventricular transmural pressure, CPAP may reduce afterload and increase cardiac output in patients with compromised left ventricular function,[24,25] making it an attractive modality for the therapy of acute pulmonary edema.

Based on the above physiologic rationale, use of CPAP (10–12.5 cm H_2O) to treat acute pulmonary edema has now been evaluated in 4 randomized controlled trials (Table 3). In a total of over 200 patients and controls, CPAP has been shown to be highly effective in avoiding intubation, reducing intubation rates from 47% among controls to 19% among CPAP-treated patients. CPAP was also highly effective in reducing respiratory rates and dyspnea scores, and in improving oxygenation, with most studies showing roughly 20–30% increases in PaO_2 or PaO_2/FiO_2 within the first hour (Table 3). Studies that have examined other outcome variables such as intensive care unit (ICU) or hospital lengths of stay, and morbidity and mortality, have shown a reduction

Table 3
Randomized Controlled Trials of CPAP in Acute Pulmonary Edema

Author	Year	Positive Pressure (cm H_2O)	No. of Patients		$PaCO_2$ (mm Hg)		$PaCO_2$ (mm Hg)	
			CPAP	Control	B	A	B	A
Rasanen et al.[24]	1985	10	20(7)	20(13)	41	39	52	60
Lin and Chiang[26]	1991	12.5	25(7)	30(18)	30	32	326	416*
Bersten et al.[27]	1991	10	19(0)	20(7)	58	46	138	206*
Lin et al.[28]	1995	12.5	50(8)	50(18)			not given	
Totals			114(22)	120(56)				
Failure rate			19%	47%				

Numbers in parentheses indicate number of failures; Failure rate: percent of patients needing intubation.
*PaO_2/FiO_2.

in ICU length of stay.[27,28] In addition, one study showed trends toward improved hospital and long-term survival.[28]

Some investigators have hypothesized that if CPAP alone is effective in the therapy of acute pulmonary edema, then NPPV (using inspiratory pressure support and PEEP) should be even better. The latter would provide the benefits of CPAP, but in addition, would provide inspiratory assistance that should further reduce inspiratory muscle work and more promptly alleviate dyspnea and gas exchange deficits, thereby improving patient tolerance. Ultimately, such benefits should more often avert respiratory failure and the need for intubation than with CPAP alone. Unfortunately, few controlled trials have evaluated the efficacy of NPPV in acute pulmonary edema, but several uncontrolled trials have been published. In their initial description of NPPV for acute respiratory failure, Meduri et al.[29] reported that 1 of 2 patients with acute pulmonary edema had an "excellent" response to NPPV. Subsequently, the same authors included 8 patients with acute pulmonary edema in their large series of patients treated with face mask PSV, 4 of whom avoided intubation.[3] Others[30] have reported small case series of patients with acute pulmonary edema treated successfully with NPPV.

More recently, 2 similar case series were reported demonstrating a low rate of intubation and few complications associated with the use of PSV plus PEEP via a face mask for acute pulmonary edema. Hoffmann et al.[31] noted only 1 intubation among 29 patients, and Rusterholtz et al.[32] observed 5 intubations among 26 patients treated with inspiratory and expiratory pressures of 17 cm H_2O and 6 cm H_2O, and

21 cm H_2O and 4 cm H_2O, respectively. Both studies observed rapid improvements in oxygen saturation and reductions in $PaCO_2$ (62 to 48 mm Hg and 54 to 43 mm Hg, respectively). Deaths occurred in 4 and 5 patients in the 2 studies, respectively, 3 and 4 of whom had myocardial infarctions. In an accompanying editorial, Wysocki noted that the use of NPPV in these patients appears to be effective, but cautioned about its use in patients with myocardial infarctions.[33]

In the only controlled trial published to date comparing CPAP (10 cm H_2O) to NPPV (using inspiratory and expiratory pressures of 15 cm H_2O and 5 cm H_2O, respectively), Mehta et al.[34] found that patients treated with NPPV had more rapid reductions in $PaCO_2$ than the CPAP group. However, myocardial infarction rate was higher (71% in the NPPV group vs. 31% in the CPAP group, p=0.06). Rates of intubation, morbidity, and mortality were similar between the 2 groups. More patients in the NPPV than in the CPAP group had chest pain upon entry into the study (10 vs. 4, p=0.06), raising questions about the adequacy of patient randomization. The authors concluded that most patients can be managed successfully with CPAP alone, but because it lowers $PaCO_2$ more rapidly than CPAP, NPPV may have advantages in patients with marked CO_2 retention on presentation. They also advised caution when applying NPPV to patients with acute cardiac ischemia or infarction and recommended that the hemodynamic effects of NPPV be further evaluated.

In a recent meta-analysis of studies on the noninvasive therapy of acute pulmonary edema, Pang et al.[35] came to the same conclusion as Mehta et al.[34] regarding CPAP, but considered the evidence on NPPV too scanty to support any conclusions. Based on the above data, CPAP should be considered the modality of first choice for patients with acute pulmonary edema. NPPV can be reserved for patients who are found to have substantial CO_2 retention or who remain dyspneic after initiation of CPAP.

Selection criteria for patients to receive noninvasive positive pressure (CPAP or NPPV) parallel those for COPD patients, but with some modifications (Table 4). First, patients should have moderate to severe respiratory distress in order to warrant assistance, but more rapid respiratory rates than COPD patients (i.e., >30–35 breaths/min). Because blood gases are not immediately available when these patients present, and $PaCO_2$ tends to be a poor indicator of the severity of respiratory distress, no firm arterial blood gas criteria are given. Caution is advised when patients have borderline blood pressures (90–100 mm Hg) because of the tendency for hemodynamic instability in these patients. Also, patients presenting with ischemic changes on the elec-

Table 4
Suggested Guidelines for Use of
Noninvasive Positive Pressure Techniques in Acute Pulmonary Edema

Selection
Clinical
  Clinical diagnosis of acute pulmonary edema
  Moderate to severe respiratory distress
  Tachypnea (RR > 30 breaths/min)
  Use of accessory muscles or abdominal paradox
Gas Exchange
  $PaO_2/FiO_2 < 300$*

Exclusion
  Comatose or respiratory arrest
  Unstable cardiac status
    Uncontrolled arrhythmias
    Acute uncontrolled ischemia
    Acute transmural myocardial infarction
    Unstable hemodynamic status
  Other exclusions as per Table 2

Techniques
  CPAP (10–12.5 cm H_2O) modality of first choice
  NPPV (11–12/5 cm H_2O inspiratory/expiratory pressures)
    If $PACO_2 > 50$ mmHg or respiratory distress persists after CPAP

*Clinical criteria are more important than gas exchange criteria; this is not a firm guideline.

trocardiogram should be monitored closely, and those with transmural infarctions who otherwise meet criteria for ventilatory assistance probably warrant intubation in view of their high risk for further hemodynamic and other complications. CPAP is recommended as the modality of first choice, but NPPV (inspiratory/expiratory pressure of 11–12/4.5 cm H_2O) may be advantageous when patients are found to be severely hypercapnic ($PaCO_2 > 50$ mm Hg) or remain dyspneic on CPAP alone.

Pneumonia

Acute pneumonia has been treated with noninvasive ventilation in a number of case series. Ambrosino et al.[36] reported a high failure rate among patients with pneumonia in their series and found a correlation between the diagnosis of pneumonia and the likelihood of NPPV failure. In their large series, Meduri et al.[3] included patients with various types of pneumonia. When pneumonia complicated COPD, the failure rate for NPPV was higher than for COPD alone (44% vs.19%). Among patients with pneumonia and no known underlying lung disease, the failure rate was 45%, and for those with AIDS-related pneumonias, only 11% required intubation.

A recent controlled trial on 56 patients with severe community-acquired pneumonia treated with face mask PSV showed avoidance of intubation in 79% of patients compared with 50% in the conventionally treated group.[37] When a subgroup analysis was performed, the benefit was seen in patients who had pneumonias complicating underlying COPD. Also, NPPV shortened the average duration of the ICU stay (9 days vs. 15 days), although total hospital length of stay and mortality rates were similar in both groups. However, much lower success rates have been reported for NPPV in pneumonia patients, with one group reporting rates as low as 10%.[38] The reasons for these differences in reported success rates are unclear, but differences in the targeted patient population, application techniques, and experience of the clinicians may have been contributing factors. The available evidence indicates that NPPV can be used successfully to treat patients with respiratory failure due to acute pneumonia, but the variable results between studies suggest that patient selection criteria are important. The studies also suggest that if a COPD patient has pneumonia, the likelihood of success with NPPV is lower than for COPD patients without pneumonia.[3] On the other hand, the pneumonia patient with COPD appears to be more likely to succeed with NPPV than a patient with respiratory failure due to acute pneumonia and no underlying lung disease.[37]

Immunocompromised patients have been considered particularly attractive candidates for NPPV because of the risk of superimposed nosocomial pneumonia and bleeding (in thrombocytopenic patients) if these patients are intubated. Along these lines, Meduri et al.[3] reported a 70% success rate with NPPV in 11 AIDS patients with Pneumocystis carinii pneumonia, and Ambrosino et al.[39] avoided intubation in 2 of 3 patients with pneumonias that developed after lung transplantation. One of these patients failed to tolerate a face mask, but was successfully managed using a poncho-wrap ventilator. More recently, Antonelli et al.[40] performed a randomized controlled trial on 40 patients with acute respiratory failure following solid organ transplantation. Of 20 patients randomized to receive face mask PSV, only 4 (20%) required intubation, as opposed to 14 (70%) of the 20 controls treated with O_2 supplementation alone (p<0.05). The PaO_2/FiO_2 ratio also improved more rapidly and fatal complications and deaths in the ICU were fewer among NPPV-treated patients. However, when an intention-to-treat analysis was used, length of ICU stay and hospital mortality (7 deaths in the NPPV-treated group compared with 11 deaths in the control group, p=0.17) were not significantly different. These studies support the use of NPPV prior to consideration of intubation for immunocompromised patients with acute pneumonias (including post-transplant, postchemotherapy neutropenia, and AIDS patients). However, the failure in the Antonelli study to show improved hospital mortality underlines the difficulty in reversing the underlying process, even if complications of mechanical ventilation are reduced.

Selection of patients with acute pneumonia to receive NPPV is complicated by the fact that many of these patients have problems expectorating secretions, and the clinician must judge whether the problem is sufficient to forego a trial of NPPV. No objective criteria have been developed to assess the quantity of secretions or impairment of the ability to protect the airway, so clinicians rely heavily on bedside observation and intuition. Otherwise, the selection process is very much like that for ARDS (Table 2). As was the case with other non-COPD causes of acute respiratory failure, clinicians are advised to be wary of prescribing NPPV for patients with acute pneumonia if the hemodynamic status is tentative. Also, if the oxygenation defect is very severe, or if the patient is developing multiorgan system failure associated with sepsis, NPPV should be avoided, because these patients are likely to have a prolonged bout of acute respiratory failure.

Other Applications of NPPV for Acute Respiratory Failure

Successful application of CPAP and NPPV has been reported in sporadic cases of other forms of acute respiratory failure, such as acute pulmonary embolism.[41,42] In addition, both CPAP and NPPV have been successfully applied to patients with trauma, including flail chest. In one study using CPAP (5–10 cm H_2O),[43] oxygenation was consistently improved, and only 2 of 33 patients (1 of 6 with flail chest) required intubation. In another study on 30 trauma or burn patients with acute hypoxemic respiratory failure treated with PSV plus PEEP (12 cm H_2O and 4 cm H_2O, respectively), respiratory rate (32 to 20 breaths/min), oxygenation, and $PaCO_2$ improved within an hour. The failure rate was 27%, with 8 patients eventually requiring intubation.[44] Unfortunately, neither of these studies was controlled, and information on the application of NPPV in trauma patients is too scanty to establish efficacy or to make recommendations on patient selection. Another application of NPPV in the acute setting has been to assist ventilation during fiberoptic bronchoscopy in immunocompromised patients at high risk of respiratory failure in whom avoidance of intubation is desirable.[45]

Hypoxemic Respiratory Failure

Studies on the use of NPPV for patients with specific non-COPD causes of acute respiratory failure have been limited by the difficulty of accumulating statistically meaningful numbers of patients, even at multiple centers. Some investigators have attempted to circumvent this problem by lumping patients into the category of "hypoxemic respiratory failure." Defined as moderate to severe respiratory distress with a PaO_2/FiO_2 ratio of < 200, this category consists of patients with a variety of causes for their acute respiratory failure, including acute pneumonia, acute pulmonary edema, ARDS, and post-trauma and postoperative patients. In their original study, Meduri et al.[29] included 4 patients with hypoxemic respiratory failure; 2 with acute pulmonary edema and 2 with acute pneumonia. All were treated successfully with NPPV. Subsequently, Wysocki et al.[46] reported on the results of NPPV therapy for patients with acute respiratory failure of non-COPD causes, some with and some without CO_2 retention. They found that 7 of 8 patients with a $PaCO_2$ < 45 mm Hg failed NPPV, whereas 7 of 9 with an initial $PaCO_2$ > 45 mm Hg were successfully treated. In a follow-up randomized trial on similar patients,[20] these same authors found no benefit of NPPV over conventional therapy among all entered patients. When patients with a $PaCO_2$ < 45 mm Hg (90% of whom required intubation) were excluded in a post hoc analysis, NPPV significantly reduced intubation rate, length of ICU stay, and ICU mortality among the remaining hypercapnic patients. The authors concluded that patients with hypoxemic respiratory failure and no CO_2 retention respond poorly to NPPV.

On the other hand, more recent uncontrolled studies suggest that some patients with hypoxemic respiratory failure may respond favorably to NPPV. Patrick et al.[19] found that NPPV using the proportional assist ventilation mode was successful in 8 of 11 patients with de novo respiratory failure who were in need of immediate intubation. Among these 8 patients were 4 with severe hypoxemia and no CO_2 retention who had rapid improvements in dyspnea scores and avoided intubation while the cause of their respiratory failure was treated. In the large series of Meduri et al.,[3] 41 of 158 patients had hypoxemic respiratory failure. This subgroup had multiple causes for their respiratory failure including COPD, pneumonia, ARDS, pulmonary edema, and restrictive lung disease. Despite having average initial PaO_2/FiO_2 ratios of 110 mm Hg, only 34% of these patients required intubation. In addition, mortality was 22% compared with a predicted mortality (using the APACHE II score) of 40%.

In a recent, controlled trial of 64 patients with hypoxemic respiratory failure randomized to receive NPPV or intubation,[47] only 31% of the NPPV-treated patients subsequently required intubation. Improvements in oxygenation were comparable in the 2 groups, and NPPV-treated patients had significantly fewer septic complications such as pneumonia or sinusitis (3% vs. 31%). In addition, NPPV-treated patients had lower mortality rates and lengths of ICU stay (27% vs. 45% and 9 days vs. 15 days, respectively), although the differences were not statistically significant.

Most recently, in a randomized controlled trial of 61 patients with various causes of respiratory failure treated with a bilevel ventilator via a nasal mask, Martin et al.[48] found that the rate of intubation was reduced from 22.6/100 ICU days among controls to 7.5/100 ICU days for NPPV-treated patients. There was also a trend for reduced mortality rate among NPPV-treated patients (2.39 vs. 4.27 deaths/100 ICU days), but the difference was not statistically significant.

Thus, although recent evidence on the use of NPPV in patients with hypoxemic respiratory failure is, for the most part, favorable, the existing data are conflicting, and further study is needed to establish efficacy and to better define ways of identifying subgroups of patients who are likely to benefit. Because the category of hypoxemic respiratory failure is a "mixed bag," it is conceivable that certain diagnoses included within it (such as acute pulmonary edema) respond favorably to NPPV, whereas others (such as ARDS or acute severe pneumonia) do not. In future studies, investigators are encouraged to focus on specific diagnostic categories so that efficacy and selection criteria can be better defined.

Summary and Conclusions

NPPV has been used to assist ventilation and avoid intubation in many forms of acute respiratory failure. Unfortunately, very few controlled trials have been performed, so efficacy remains unestablished and selection of patients is based on experience and guesswork rather than on validated criteria. The one diagnostic category in which controlled data have accrued from multiple trials is acute cardiogenic pulmonary edema, but this is for CPAP rather than NPPV. Accordingly,

CPAP is considered the ventilatory mode of first choice for pulmonary edema patients. For the other categories, NPPV can be tried before consideration of intubation, but only in carefully selected patients. In addition to choosing patients with moderate to severe respiratory distress, clinicians must be especially careful to exclude patients who are at higher risk if intubation is inappropriately delayed. Deciding when patients have "excessive" secretions, "inability " to protect the airway, or are too uncooperative is a clinical skill that requires judgment and experience. Even in the best hands, however, noninvasive ventilation fails in 20–40% of cases, and those with non-COPD causes would be expected to occupy the higher levels of this range. When in doubt, a brief trial of NPPV could be undertaken, but the prudent clinician should be prepared to intubate the patient after 1 or 2 hours without improvement.

References

1. Meduri GU, Abou-Shala N, Fox RC, et al. Noninvasive face mask mechanical ventilation in patients with acute hypercapnic respiratory failure. Chest 1991;100:445-454.
2. Pennock BE, Kaplan PD, Carlin BW, et al. Pressure support ventilation with a simplified ventilatory support system administered with a nasal mask in patients with respiratory failure. Chest 1991;100:1371-1376.
3. Meduri GU, Turner RE, Abou-Shala N, et al. Noninvasive positive pressure ventilation via face mask. Chest 1996;109:179-193.
4. Meduri GU, Cook TR, Turner RE, et al. Noninvasive positive pressure ventilation in status asthmaticus. Chest 1996;110:767-774.
5. Weiss EB, Faling LF. Clinical significance of $PaCO_2$ during status asthma. Ann Allergy 1968;26:545-553.
6. Hill NS, Weiss EB. Status asthmaticus. In Weiss EB, Stein M (eds). Bronchial Asthma, Mechanisms and Therapeutics. 3rd Ed. Boston, MA, Little Brown, 1993, pp 985-1016.
7. Skobeloff EM, Spivey WH, McNamara RM, et al. Intravenous magnesium suflate for the treatment of acute asthma in the emergency department. JAMA 1989;262:1210-1213.
8. Kass JE, Terregino CA. The effect of heliox in acute severe asthma: a randomized controlled trial. Chest 1999;116:296-300.
9. Pollack CV Jr, Fleisch KB, Dowsey K. Treatment of acute bronchospasm with beta-adrenergic agonist aerosols delivered by a nasal bilevel positive airway pressure circuit. Ann Emerg Med 1995;26:552-557.
10. Murray JF. Review of the state of the art in intermittent positive pressure breathing therapy. Am Rev Respir Dis 1974;110:193-203.
11. Hodson ME, Madden BP, Steven MH, et al. Noninvasive mechanical ventilation for cystic fibrosis patients: a potential bridge to transplantation. Eur Respir J 1991;4:524-527.

12. Sturani C, Galavotti V, Scarduelli C, et al. Acute respiratory failure due to severe obstructive sleep apnoea syndrome, managed with nasal positive pressure ventilation. Monaldi Arch Chest Dis 1994;49:558-560.
13. Piper AJ, Sullivan CE. Sleep-disordered breathing in neuromuscular disease. In Saunders NA, Sullivan CE (eds). Sleeping and Breathing. 2nd Ed. New York, Marcel Dekker, Inc., 1994, pp 761-786.
14. Bach JR. Conventional approaches to managing neuromuscular ventilatory failure. In Bach JR (ed). Pulmonary Rehabilitation: The Obstructive and Paralytic Conditions. Philadelphia, Henley & Belfus, 1996, pp 285-301.
15. Finlay G, Concannon D, McDonell TJ. Treatment of respiratory failure due to kyphoscoliosis with nasal intermittent positive pressure ventilation (NIPPV). Irish J Med Sci 1995;164:28-30.
16. Bach JR, Ishikawa Y, Kim H. Prevention of pulmonary morbidity for patients with Duchenne muscular dystrophy. Chest 1997;112:1024-1028.
17. Bach JR. Mechanical insufflation-exsufflation: comparison of peak expiratory flows with manually assisted and unassisted coughing techniques. Chest 1993;104:1553-1564.
18. Bach JR. Update and perspective on noninvasive respiratory muscle aids. Part 2: The expiratory aids. Chest 1994;105:1538-1544.
19. Patrick W, Webster K, Ludwig L, et al. Noninvasive positive pressure ventilation. I. Acute respiratory distress without prior chronic respiratory failure. Am J Respir Crit Care Med 1996;153:1005-1011.
20. Wysocki M, Laurent T, Wolff MA, et al. Noninvasive pressure support ventilation in patients with acute respiratory failure: a randomized comparison with conventional therapy. Chest 1995;107:761-768.
21. Rocker GM, Mackensie MG, Williams B, Logan PM. Noninvasive positive pressure ventilation: successful outcome in patients with acute lung injury/ARDS. Chest 1999;115:173-177.
22. Barach AL, Martin J, Eckman M. Positive pressure respiration and its application to the treatment of acute pulmonary edema. Ann Intern Med 1938;12:754-795.
23. Katz JA, Marks JD. Inspiratory work with and without continuous positive airway pressure in patients with acute respiratory failure. Anesthesiology 1985;63:598-607.
24. Rasanen J, Vaisanen IT, Heikkila J, et al. Acute myocardial infarction complicated by left ventricular dysfunction and respiratory failure. Chest 1985;87:158-162.
25. Fessler HR, Brower R, Wise R, et al. Effects of systolic and diastolic positive pleural pressure on cardiac output with altered cardiac contractility. Am Rev Respir Dis 1988;137:293.
26. Lin M, Chiang H. The efficacy of early continuous positive airway pressure therapy in patients with acute cardiogenic pulmonary edema. J Formosan Med Assoc 1991;90:736-743.
27. Bersten AD, Holt AW, Vedig AE, et al. Treatment of severe cardiogenic pulmonary edema with continuous positive airway pressure delivered by face mask. N Engl J Med 1991;325:1825-1830.
28. Lin M, Yang Y, Chiany H, et al. Reappraisal of continuous positive airway pressure therapy in acute cardiogenic pulmonary edema: short-term results and long-term follow-up. Chest 1995;107:1379-1386.

29. Meduri GU, Conoscenti CC, Menashe P, et al. Noninvasive face mask ventilation in patients with acute respiratory failure. Chest 1989;95:865-870.
30. Lapinsky SE, Mount DNB, Mackey D, et al. Management of acute respiratory failure due to pulmonary edema with nasal positive pressure support. Chest 1994;105:229-231.
31. Hoffmann B, Welte T. The use of noninvasive pressure support ventilation for severe respiratory insufficiency due to pulmonary oedema. Intensive Care Med 1999;25:15-20.
32. Rusterholtz T, Kempf J, Berton C, et al. Noninvasive pressure support ventilation (NIPSV) with face mask in patients with acute cardiogenic pulmonary edema (ACPE). Intensive Care Med 1999;25:21-28.
33. Wysocki M. Being more positive about negative ventilation? Eur Respir J 1998;12:515-516.
34. Mehta S, Jay GD, Woolard RH, et al. Randomized prospective trial of bilevel versus continuous positive airway pressure in acute pulmonary edema. Crit Care Med 1997;25:620-628.
35. Pang D, Keenan SP, Cook DJ, Sibbald WJ. The effect of positive pressure airway support on mortality and the need for intubation in cardiogenic pulmonary edema. Chest 1998;114:1185-1192.
36. Ambrosino N, Foglio K, Rubini F, et al. Noninvasive mechanical ventilation in acute respiratory failure due to chronic obstructive pulmonary disease: correlates for success. Thorax 1995;50:755-757.
37. Confalonieri M, Potena A, Carbone G, et al. Acute respiratory failure in patients with severe community-acquired pneumonia. Am J Respir Crit Care Med 1999;160:1585-1591.
38. Averill FJ, Adkins G. Use of bilevel positive airway pressure (BiPAP) in patients with acute respiratory failure. Chest 1993;104:143S.
39. Ambrosino N, Rubini F, Callegari G, et al. Noninvasive mechanical ventilation in the treatment of acute respiratory failure due to infectious complications of lung transplantation. Monaldi Arch Chest Dis 1994;49:311-314.
40. Antonelli M, Conti C, Bufi M, et al. Noninvasive ventilation for treatment of acute respiratory failure in patients undergoing solid organ transplantation. JAMA 2000;283:235-241.
41. Orta DA, Tucker NH, Green LE, et al. Severe hypoxemia secondary to pulmonary embolization treated successfully with the use of a CPAP (continuous positive airway pressure) mask. Chest 1978;74:588-590.
42. Kramer N, Meyer TJ, Meharg J, et al. Randomized, prospective trial of noninvasive positive pressure ventilation in acute respiratory failure. Am J Respir Crit Care Med 1995;151:1799-1806.
43. Hurst JM, DeHaven CB, Branson RD. Use of CPAP mask as the sole mode of ventilatory support in trauma patients with mild to moderate respiratory insufficiency. J Trauma 1985;25:1065-1068.
44. Gregoretti C, Beltrame F, Lucangelo U, et al. Physiologic evaluation of noninvasive pressure support ventilation in trauma patients with acute respiratory failure. Intensive Care Med 1998;24:785-790.
45. Antonelli M, Conti G, Riccioni L, Meduri GU. Noninvasive positive-pressure ventilation via face mask during bronchoscopy with BAL in high-risk hypoxemic patients. Chest 1996;110:724-728.

46. Wysocki M, Tric L, Wolff MA, et al. Noninvasive pressure support ventilation in patients with acute respiratory failure. Chest 1993;107:761-768.
47. Antonelli M, Conti G, Rocco M, et al. A comparison of noninvasive positive pressure ventilation with conventional mechanical ventilation in patients with acute respiratory failure. N Engl J Med 1998;339:429–435.
48. Martin TJ, Hovis JD, Constantino JP, et al. A randomized, prospective evaluation of noninvasive ventilation for acute respiratory failure. Am J Respir Crit Care Med 2000;161:807-813.

Chapter 6

Other Applications of Noninvasive Positive Pressure Ventilation in the Acute Care Setting

Nicholas S. Hill, M.D.

Introduction

The previous two chapters have addressed the application of noninvasive positive pressure ventilation (NPPV) for acute respiratory failure in patients with various diagnoses of respiratory disease. NPPV is also used in several clinical scenarios in the acute setting, with the specific diagnosis becoming a secondary consideration. These include patients with postoperative respiratory insufficiency, those who have declined intubation, and those who are weaning from invasive mechanical ventilation. Each of these will now be discussed, with consideration of the evidence supporting the application, and provision of patient selection guidelines.

Postoperative Patients

Patients who develop respiratory insufficiency after surgery are at risk for further complications, including the need for intubation (or reintubation) and prolonged invasive mechanical ventilation. By stabilizing patients and averting the need for intubation, NPPV may lower the complication rates and shorten the hospital lengths of stay. Pennock et al.[1] were the first to study this potential application of NPPV. Using nasal ventilation via a BiPAP device, these authors prevented the need for reintubation in 19 of 24 patients who had respiratory deteriorations at least 36 hours following various types of surgery. To be enrolled, these patients had to have a $PaCO_2 > 50$ mm Hg, $PaO_2 < 60$ mm Hg, or evidence of respiratory muscle fatigue. In response to

From *Noninvasive Positive Pressure Ventilation: Principles and Applications,* edited by Nicholas S. Hill. © 2001, Futura Publishing Company, Inc., Armonk, NY.

1 hour of NPPV in these patients, respiratory rate dropped from 30 breaths/min to 23 breaths/min, $PaCO_2$ fell from 49 mm Hg to 44 mm Hg, PaO_2 rose from 74 mm Hg to 91 mm Hg, and dyspnea scores (Borg scale) fell from 6.5 to 1.5. In a follow-up study[2] on 110 patients, 80% of whom were postoperative, these authors found that this initial success rate was sustained, even when NPPV was administered as a "usual care" procedure rather than as a special research technique.

More recently, Aguilo et al.[3] tested the idea that NPPV could be used prophylactically to maintain improved gas exchange in postoperative patients who are at risk for respiratory complications. After lung resection, they randomized 19 patients to receive nasal "bilevel" ventilation (inspiratory pressure, 10 cm H_2O; expiratory pressure, 5 cm H_2O) or routine care soon after they were extubated. During a 1-hour trial, PaO_2 improved more in the NPPV group compared with controls (78 mm Hg vs. 69 mm Hg), and no adverse side effects were encountered. Testing the same possibility in morbidly obese patients after gastroplasty, Joris et al.[4] found that 1 day of BiPAP via a face mask at inspiratory and expiratory pressures of 12 cm H_2O and 4 cm H_2O, respectively, significantly reduced the pulmonary dysfunction that follows gastroplasty. More recently, Munshi et al.[5] evaluated the outcomes of bilevel ventilation in 536 patients extubated after surgery. Thirteen were reintubated immediately for severe respiratory failure or inspiratory stridor, but 72 others were hypoxemic and were treated with NPPV. The authors concluded that NPPV could be used to reduce the need for oxygen supplementation in postoperative patients, resulting in a cost savings. Of these, 72% improved and 28% failed. Of course, lacking randomized controls, the efficacy of NPPV using bilevel ventilation relative to continuous positive airway pressure (CPAP) or O_2 supplementation alone cannot be ascertained in the above studies. These studies demonstrate that NPPV can be used to improve gas exchange and pulmonary function in postoperative patients, but further controlled trials are needed to establish whether these benefits are truly prophylactic, translating into other improved outcomes such as reduced intubation, morbidity or mortality rates, or shorter lengths of stay.

Criteria for selection of postoperative patients to receive NPPV have not been established, but most authors have used criteria similar to those for patients presenting with acute respiratory failure in a nonsurgical setting (Table 1). Because the use is prophylactic, the guidelines aim to identify at-risk patients, based on premorbid cardiopulmonary disease, and the risk of the surgical procedures. Thus, those with known histories of severe obstructive or restrictive disease, or underlying congestive heart failure, or those who have undergone major chest

Table 1
Suggested Guidelines for
Prophylactic Use of NPPV in High Risk Postoperative Patients

Clinical
Risk Factors
  High risk diagnosis
    Severe COPD
    Obstructive sleep apnea
    Morbid obesity
    Restrictive thoracic disorder
    Congestive heart failure
  High risk procedure
    Lung resection
    Lung transplantation
    Upper abdominal procedure
    Gastroplasty
    Major chest or abdominal procedure
  Postoperative respiratory deterioration
    Increased respiratory distress
    Tachypnea (RR > 24 breaths/min)
    Accessory muscle use
    Abdominal paradox
  Gas Exchange
    Increasing $PaCO_2$ (> 45 mm Hg)
    Decreasing $PaCO_2$ (< 60 mm Hg) or PaO_2/FiO_2 < 200)
Exclusions
  Respiratory arrest
  Other medical instability (uncontrolled cardiac arrhythmias, ischemia, or upper
    GI bleeding)
  Uncooperative
  Unable to protect airway or control secretions
  Head, neck or upper airway/esophageal surgery

or abdominal procedures would receive prophylactic NPPV if they manifested respiratory distress or gas exchange deterioration during the postoperative period. The exclusions are the same as those for other applications of NPPV, except that more attention must be paid to the nature of the surgical procedure. Those with recent upper airway or esophageal procedures should not receive NPPV, and most recipients of head and neck surgery will not be able to accommodate a mask.

As discussed above, the prophylactic use of NPPV in postoperative patients shows promise but has not yet been shown to improve outcomes other than physiologic ones. Nonetheless, the studies provide a rationale for the early application of NPPV in high risk patients, such as the morbidly obese, or those with severe underlying lung disease or moderate oxygenation defects, before the occurrence of a significant deterioration in respiratory status.

Do-Not-Intubate Patients

Many patients with severe lung disease or other potentially terminal conditions decline intubation in the event of a severe deterioration. Some of these patients are still willing to try NPPV, even though they continue to refuse invasive ventilation. Benhamou et al.[6] studied 30 such patients, most elderly with chronic obstructive pulmonary disease (COPD), in whom endotracheal intubation was "contraindicated or postponed." Despite severe respiratory failure (mean initial pH, 7.29; PaO_2, 44 mm Hg; $PaCO_2$, 65 mm Hg), 18 (60%) of cases were successfully supported and weaned. Seven patients were intolerant of the ventilator, and 12 eventually failed, with 8 dying and 4 requiring "postponed" endotracheal intubation. In another uncontrolled series, Meduri et al.[7] observed a similar response to NPPV among 11 patients with acute hypercapnic (9 patients) or hypoxemic (2 patients) respiratory failure who refused intubation. Short-term success rate was 64%, and 45% of patients survived the hospitalization. In their randomized, controlled trial on acute exacerbations in 60 COPD patients, Bott et al.[8] used invasive mechanical ventilation in only 1 of the 9 control patients (of 30) who died. Of the 30 patients randomized to receive NPPV, only 3 died. Thus, the survival advantage they observed among NPPV-treated patients was, in effect, in comparison to do-not-intubate patients.

Based on these findings, the use of NPPV for patients who are not to receive invasive ventilation is justifiable as long as the patient understands that NPPV is a form of life support, albeit noninvasive, and there is some prospect for reversal of the acute process. Ideally, ventilatory options should be discussed with the patient and family well in advance of the onset of a respiratory crisis, but decisions often have to be made at the time of the acute hospitalization. One could argue that there is little to lose by using NPPV in almost any terminal patient. In fact, some have described the use of NPPV as a palliative intervention, providing a few hours to days of extended survival in terminally ill patients, to allow time for completion of end-of-life issues.[9] It could also be argued that it is humane to use NPPV for alleviation of dyspnea in a terminal patient, in essence as a mechanical narcotic. However, these latter applications are highly controversial, with others arguing that indiscriminate use of NPPV should be discouraged, be-

Table 2
Suggested Guidelines for Use
of NPPV in Patients Who Decline Intubation

Selection Guidelines
  Clinical
    Moderate to severe respiratory distress
    Tachypnea (> 24–30 breaths/min)
    Use of accessory muscles or abdominal paradox
  Gas Exchange
    Increasing hypercapnia ($PaCO_2$ > 45 mm Hg) or
    Deteriorating oxygenation (PaO_2/FiO_2 < 200)
Exclusions
  No chance of reversal of process
  Copious uncontrolled secretions
  Marked agitation, unresponsive to sedation

cause this could merely prolong the dying process and lead to inappropriate resource utilization.[10]

Considering that the do-not-intubate patient has no other option for ventilatory assistance besides noninvasive ventilation, selection criteria can be liberalized (Table 2). NPPV can be tried in patients with excessive secretions, impaired swallowing or cough, or unresponsiveness, and sometimes patients with severe CO_2 narcosis will awaken as their $PaCO_2$ falls. On the other hand, exclusion of patients should be considered if there is no chance of reversal and the use of NPPV is likely to be futile. Thus, patients with end-stage malignancy, marked agitation, or severe secretion retention have a sufficiently low likelihood of success that use of NPPV should be discouraged.

Facilitation of Weaning and Extubation

Noninvasive Ventilation for Early Extubation

Patients with acute respiratory failure who are not candidates for NPPV and who require intubation when they are initially admitted to the hospital may rapidly stabilize and become candidates for noninvasive ventilation within a few days. If such patients encounter difficulty with weaning, early removal of the endotracheal tube and initiation of NPPV could reduce complications of prolonged intubation such as nosocomial infection and upper airway trauma. As long as the patient has an intact cough mechanism, early removal of the tube permits restoration of the normal airway defense mechanisms, including cough and mucociliary clearance. Pooling of secretions above the endotracheal tube cuff is also eliminated, removing a potentially dangerous source of lower airway contamination. In addition, removal of the tube would lower upper airway resistance related to the presence of the tube. These and other potential advantages of early tube removal are listed in Table 3.

The first use of NPPV to facilitate extubation was reported by Udwadia et al.[11] who studied 22 consecutive patients with difficult weaning. Most of the patients had hypercapnic respiratory insufficiency, 9 with chest wall defects, 6 with neuromuscular disorders, and 7 with cardiac disease. All had failed at least one weaning attempt, and were considered candidates for NPPV if they had intact bulbar function with a preserved cough reflex, minimal airway secretions, the ability to breathe spontaneously for 10–15 minutes, low oxygen supplementation requirements, cardiac stability, and a functioning gastrointestinal tract. Patients were treated initially with nasal mask ventilation for 16–20 hours per 24 hours and then gradually weaned to nocturnal use, depending on the rate of individual patient recovery. Twenty patients made successful transitions to noninvasive ventilation and were transferred from the intensive care unit (ICU) to a step-down unit or a general ward. The 2 patients who failed had pulmonary fibrosis. The average duration of invasive ventilation was 31 days, but some patients had been treated invasively for more than 200 days. The average duration of noninvasive ventilation was only approximately 10% of the duration of invasive ventilation (Figure 1), and all successfully weaned patients improved rapidly once they had been switched

Table 3
Potential Advantages and Disadvantages of Early Endotracheal Tube Removal

Potential Advantages	Disadvantages
Improves patient comfort	Loss of direct airway access
Restores normal speech	No endotracheal suctioning
Restores normal eating	Less ability to sedate agitated patients
Restores cough mechanism	Discomfort related to mask
Mucociliary clearance restored	Less assured ventilatory assistance
Sinus drainage restored (if nasal tubes removed)	Possible increase in extubation failure rates
Reduces nosocomial infection rates	
Reduces mortality	

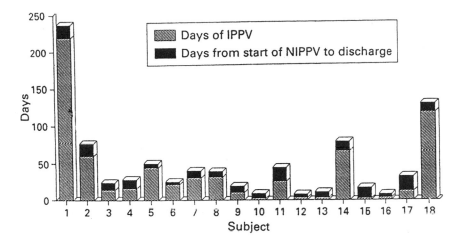

Figure 1. Number of days patients received invasive intermittent positive pressure ventilation (IPPV) and the number of days from the start of noninvasive ventilation (NIPPV) until hospital discharge. (From reference 11, with permission).

to noninvasive ventilation. Follow-up for an average of 21 months after discharge revealed that 16 patients were alive and well. These authors originated the idea that NPPV can be used to facilitate the weaning process, but acknowledged that the lack of controls was an important limitation.

Restrick et al.[12] subsequently reported another case series of 14 patients with findings similar to those of Udwadia et al.[11] Eight patients had COPD, 4 had restrictive disease, and 13 of the 14 patients were successfully weaned using NPPV. The patients had been intubated for differing periods of time; 3 had been intubated for only 1 day. With patients intubated for such a short period of time, this study can be credited with introducing the concept that NPPV could be started earlier than otherwise would be the case, to reduce the duration of intubation. The authors also included patients who had self-extubated prematurely, illustrating another new application of NPPV. Once again, however, the lack of controls limited the conclusions that could be drawn from this study.

The need for controlled trials was recently addressed by Nava et al.,[13] who tested the hypothesis that early extubation to NPPV could improve outcomes of patients who would otherwise have remained intubated. Sixty-eight COPD patients who had been intubated for acute respiratory failure were screened. These patients were sedated and managed with volume-limited ventilation for the first 6–12 hours and pressure support ventilation for the subsequent 24–36 hours. Forty-eight hours after intubation, if the patient was hemodynamically stable, had a normal temperature, an acceptable neurologic status, and no signs of pneumonia, a T-piece trial was performed. The 50 patients who failed the T-piece trial were randomized to extubation and to receive immediate noninvasive ventilation or to continue conventional weaning with the endotracheal tube in place. Both groups were weaned by daily reductions in the level of pressure support and spontaneous breathing trials at least twice a day. Compared with the 25 patients who remained intubated, the 25 patients randomized to receive NPPV had higher overall weaning rates (88% vs. 68%) after 60 days and shorter durations of mechanical ventilation (10.2 days vs. 16.6 days). They also had briefer stays in the ICU (15.1 days vs. 24 days) and improved 60-day survival rates (92% vs. 72%) (NPPV-treated vs. controls, all p<0.05). In addition, no NPPV-treated patients had nosocomial pneumonia, compared with 7 of the controls.

More recently, Girault et al.[14] performed a second randomized, controlled trial to address the question of whether NPPV should be used as a "systematic" extubation technique. This study randomized 33 patients with acute-on-chronic respiratory failure to receive NPPV or to remain intubated after they failed a weaning trial. Not surprisingly, the authors found that the NPPV group had a significantly shorter duration of invasive mechanical ventilation (4.56 days vs. 7.69 days, p<0.05), but the total duration of mechanical ventilation (including NPPV) was actually greater in the NPPV group (16.1 days vs. 7.69 days, p=0.0001). Further, patients in the NPPV group had similar eventual weaning and mortality rates, and although they had a tendency toward fewer complications than controls (16 vs. 9), the difference was not statistically significant. The authors concluded that NPPV shortens the duration of invasive mechanical ventilation and anticipated that this would reduce morbidity, despite the fact that they were unable to demonstrate a significant reduction in complication rates in their study.

Studies examining the use of NPPV for the early extubation of non-COPD patients with acute respiratory failure have been few. One uncontrolled study compared blood gases, tidal volumes, and respiratory rates in a group of trauma patients with hypoxemic respiratory failure at equal levels of pressure support before and after extubation.[15] After an average of 4 days of invasive ventilation, 22 trauma patients underwent a T-piece trial of at least 15 minutes and were then switched to noninvasive ventilation. Although NPPV initially maintained tidal volumes and respiratory rates as well as invasive ventilation, 9 patients

(41%) eventually required reintubation because of clinical deterioration, mask intolerance, or an inability to clear secretions, and 6 of these patients later died while still being ventilated. This study was not specifically designed to test the efficacy of NPPV as an extubation technique, but it was the first to evaluate this approach in patients without COPD or restrictive thoracic disease. Success rates were lower than in patients with acute-on-chronic respiratory failure, consistent with earlier trials showing lower success rates for NPPV in patients with non-COPD causes of respiratory failure. Thus, these findings suggest that the underlying pathology may be important in determining the outcome of early extubation.

A more recent trial evaluated the physiologic effects of CPAP (5 cm H_2O) and pressure support ventilation (15 cm H_2O) compared with spontaneous breathing in 15 non-COPD patients. These patients were mainly transplant recipients who had been extubated early after a bout of acute respiratory failure.[16] Both CPAP and pressure support improved oxygenation and shunt fraction, increased tidal volume, and lowered respiratory rate, with pressure support effecting greater improvements than CPAP alone. Only 2 of the 15 patients required intubation. The authors concluded that NPPV is a "feasible" therapeutic option in non-COPD patients with acute respiratory failure, but that more controlled trials are needed. Another recent preliminary study on the feasibility of early extubation in medical ICU patients with various causes for their acute respiratory failure found that the duration of invasive ventilation was shortened by early extubation to NPPV.[17] However, neither the total duration of ventilation nor the length of ICU or hospital stay were shortened, morbidity and mortality rates were not improved, and the extubation failure rate was significantly increased (to 43%) compared with controls.

Although the above studies are generally supportive of the use of NPPV to expedite extubation and shorten the duration of invasive ventilation in selected patients with acute-on-chronic respiratory failure (COPD or restrictive) who require initial invasive ventilation for acute respiratory failure, clinicians are encouraged to be cautious when using this approach. Favorable effects on lengths of ICU stay, weaning, and morbidity and mortality rates were seen in the Nava et al. study.[13] However, these favorable effects were not confirmed in the Girault et al.[14] study which found that early extubation to NPPV shortened the duration of invasive mechanical ventilation, but did not significantly affect other outcome variables. Thus, further trials are needed not only to confirm the Nava findings, but also to determine whether non-COPD patients may benefit, and to better define patient selection criteria.

Pending these further investigations, candidates for early extubation should be selected with extreme care. Patients who fail standard weaning trials often have comorbidities and are deconditioned, with impaired coughing abilities. If such patients are not entirely stable hemodynamically or are incapable of cooperating or expectorating secretions adequately, they are at high risk for failure while using NPPV. The concern is that overly zealous use of NPPV for early extubation may lead to an increase in the extubation failure rate, as was suggested in the trials reporting extubation failure rates of 42%[15] and 43%.[17] Epstein et al.[18] have shown that extubation failure is associated with a 7-fold increase in the risk of mortality (approximately 40%) compared with successfully extubated patients. Thus, the inappropriate use of NPPV to facilitate extubation could pose an increased risk of morbidity or mortality.

Possible criteria to be used for early extubation are listed in Table 4, but it should be borne in mind that the approach is not yet widely accepted as a standard of care. In essence, the guidelines aim to identify

---

Table 4

Suggested Guidelines for Selection
of Patients to Undergo Early Extubation to NPPV

Preferred diagnoses
  Acute on chronic hypercapnic respiratory failure
    COPD
    Restrictive thoracic disorder
Passes screen for weanability
  Arousable; not requiring continuous sedation
  Adequate oxygenation; $PaO_2 \geq 60$ mm Hg on $FiO_2 \leq 40\%$ with PEEP ≤ 5
  Intact cough
  Hemodynamically stable
Fails T-piece trial
  RR ≥ 35/min
  HR > 140/min
  Systolic BP < 90 or > 200 mm Hg
  O_2 sat $< 88\%$ on 40% FiO_2
  $PaCO_2$ increases ($> 20\%$ over hypercapnic baseline)
Good candidate for NPPV
  No need for frequent suctioning ($<$ once/hour)
  Cooperative
  Able to fit mask
Safeguards/Cautions
  Able to breathe spontaneously on T-piece > 5 min
  No copious secretions
  Not a difficult intubation

patients who fail a T-piece trial and hence would not be extubated by standard criteria, but are otherwise good candidates for NPPV. In particular, patients should have an intact cough reflex and not have excessive secretions. The latter has not been well defined, but if the patient requires frequent suctioning (i.e., more than once per hr), then early extubation should not be undertaken. Further, as a safeguard, patients should be able to breathe spontaneously using a T-piece for at least 5 minutes to allow for time for initiating NPPV once the patient is extubated. Also, if the initial intubation was difficult, caution is advised.

Noninvasive Ventilation to Facilitate Removal of a Tracheostomy Tube

The concept of using NPPV to facilitate removal of a tracheostomy tube is essentially the same as that for early removal of a translaryngeal endotracheal tube, but there is an important difference. The tracheostomy tube can be plugged and left in place during initiation of NPPV trials, and the patient can easily resume tracheostomy ventilation should problems arise. This adds a margin of safety because the patient does not have to be decannulated until it is clear that NPPV will be effective. Goodenberger et al.[19] were the first to demonstrate efficacy for this application of NPPV in a report on 2 patients with neuromuscular disease. By using NPPV nocturnally during plugging of the tube, the patients were transitioned to full NPPV, and the tracheostomy tube was removed after a period of days.

Other encouraging preliminary results have been reported by Laier-Groeneveld et al.[20] in Germany who demonstrated that, once they were switched to noninvasive ventilation, all but 1 of their 35 patients were able to undergo successful decannulation after an average of 66 days of invasive mechanical ventilation. These patients had chronic hypercapnic respiratory failure and were considered unweanable by the attending physicians. Most continued to receive nocturnal ventilatory assistance after decannulation, but remained stable with NPPV.

The above studies support the use of NPPV to facilitate removal of a tracheostomy tube, but in the absence of controlled trials, any recommendations must be tentative. Acceptable candidates would be those who are making progress with regard to recovery from underlying organ failure, have recovered the ability to cough and swallow, do not require frequent suctioning for removal of secretions, and are capable of at least some ventilator-free breathing (some authors have suggested

15 min).[10] A systematic approach to the decannulation process has been described by Viroslav et al.[21]

Avoidance of Reintubation after Extubation Failure

Another potential application of NPPV in the weaning process is to avoid reintubation in patients who fail extubation. Extubation failure occurs in 3–19% of patients after planned extubations,[18] and in 40–50% after unplanned extubations.[22] In a prospective cohort of 289 consecutive intubated patients who underwent a trial of extubation, Epstein et al.[18] observed a reintubation rate of 15%, with a mortality of 43% among those failing extubation as opposed to 12% in those who succeeded. After adjustments for severity of illness and comorbid conditions, extubation failure was associated with a 7-fold increase in the risk of death and a 31-fold increase in the likelihood of an ICU stay exceeding 14 days. Although at least part of the increase in mortality associated with extubation failure is attributable to greater pre-extubation morbidity in patients who fail compared with those who succeed, some of the morbidity and mortality may be related to the complications of reintubation and the prolongation of invasive ventilation. To the extent that this is the case, use of NPPV to reduce the need for reintubation could improve the outcome of patients who fail extubation.

Several case series and one historically controlled trial have reported success for this application of NPPV.[23,24] Meduri et al.[23] included 39 patients with postextubation respiratory failure in their series[24] of 158 patients, 65% of whom avoided reintubation. Another recent series found that 30 COPD patients with postextubation hypercapnic respiratory insufficiency required reintubation less often (20% vs. 67%) and had shorter ICU lengths of stay (18 days vs. 14 days) than 30 historically matched controls. The only randomized, prospective trial yet published on the use of noninvasive ventilation to prevent reintubation in patients after extubation enrolled 56 consecutive patients after planned, and 37 after unplanned, extubations.[25] Thirteen (28%) of the 47 patients randomized to receive "bilevel" ventilation (inspiratory pressure 12 cm H_2O, expiratory pressure 5 cm H_2O) required reintubation, compared with 7 (15%) of the 46 patients receiving O_2 supplementation alone (p> 0.05). Of the 20 total patients who failed, 14 had unplanned extubations. The most common reason for failure was excessive secretions. The authors concluded that their results did not support the "indiscriminate" use of NPPV to avoid postextubation failure.

Despite the disappointing results of this trial, it is important to consider that patients in the trial were randomized without any attempt to select those at risk for extubation failure. Pending information from further studies, a trial of NPPV for extubation failure is still an option as long as patients are carefully screened. Patients who develop inspiratory stridor soon after extubation are probably good candidates, because this condition is often reversible within hours. Noninvasive ventilation can be used to assist breathing while inflammation and swelling of the glottus subside. On the other hand, because secretion retention is a common reason for failure, attention should be paid to the volume of secretions and adequacy of cough. Patients deemed to have excessive secretions should be promptly reintubated. In general, recommendations for the selection of patients with extubation failure (Table 5) are similar to those for patients presenting with acute respiratory failure, as discussed in Chapters 4 and 5.

Table 5
Suggested Guidelines for Application
of NPPV to Patients with Extubation Failure

Clinical
Increasing dyspnea or tachypnea after extubation (> 30/min for restrictive or hypoxemic processes) or
Use of accessory muscles or abdominal paradox
Gas Exchange
Increasing $PaCO_2$ (> 45 mm Hg or > 20% over pre-extubation value) or
$PaO_2/FiO_2 \leq 200$
Preferred Diagnosis
COPD
Congestive heart failure
Upper airway obstruction (due to laryngeal or glottic edema)
Contraindications
Complete upper airway obstruction
Respiratory arrest
Excessive secretions
Unable to protect airway (impaired swallowing or cough)
Uncooperative
Medically unstable
Unable to fit mask

Summary and Conclusions

Although the use of noninvasive ventilation for patients with certain forms of acute respiratory failure such as that caused by COPD exacerbations is becoming standard therapy, for many other applications, it is not yet supported by multiple controlled trials. Such is the case for the applications discussed in this chapter. For postoperative patients who develop respiratory insufficiency, uncontrolled trials or controlled trials that have examined only physiologic outcome variables support the use of NPPV. Accordingly, although this application cannot be considered standard therapy, a trial of NPPV may be considered as long as patients are carefully selected. The use of NPPV to prevent postoperative complications shows promise, but more studies are needed to establish its efficacy. Randomized, controlled trials of NPPV for do-not-intubate patients are unlikely to be performed because of the ethical issues such studies raise. This application is supported by cohort series and is appropriate in patients with a reasonable chance of reversal of the underlying process. Its use in patients with irreversible conditions who are unlikely to survive the hospitalization is more questionable, however.

Several recent controlled trials support the use of NPPV to facilitate weaning of COPD patients from invasive mechanical ventilation. Once again, this application should be reserved for carefully selected patients. More studies are needed to examine the utility of this approach for non-COPD patients and for those who have failed extubation.

References

1. Pennock BE, Kaplan PD, Carlin BW, et al. Pressure support ventilation with a simplified ventilatory support system administered with a nasal mask in patients with respiratory failure. Chest 1991;100:1371-1376.
2. Pennock BE, Crawshaw L, Kaplan PD. Noninvasive nasal mask ventilation for acute respiratory failure. Chest 1994;105:441-444.
3. Aguilo R, Togores B, Pons S, et al. Noninvasive ventilator support after lung resectional surgery. Chest 1997;112:117-121.
4. Joris JL, Sottiaux TM, Chiche JD, et al. Effect of bilevel positive airway pressure (BiPAP) nasal ventilation on the postoperative pulmonary restrictive syndrome in obese patients undergoing gastroplasty. Chest 1997;111:665-670.
5. Munshi IA, DeHaven B, Kirton O, et al. Reengineering respiratory support following extubation avoidance of critical care unit costs. Chest 1999;116:1025-1028.
6. Benhamou D, Girault C, Faure C, et al. Nasal mask ventilation in acute respiratory failure: experience in elderly patients. Chest 1992;102:912-917.
7. Meduri GU, Fox RC, Abou-Shala N, et al. Noninvasive mechanical ventilation via face mask in patients with acute respiratory failure who refused endotracheal intubation. Crit Care Med 1994;22:1584-1590.
8. Bott J, Carroll MP, Conway JH, et al. Randomized controlled trial of nasal ventilation in acute ventilatory failure due to chronic obstructive airways disease. Lancet 1993;341:1555-1557.

9. Freichels TA. Palliative ventilatory support: use of noninvasive positive pressure ventilation in terminal respiratory insufficiency. Am J Crit Care 1994;3:6-10.
10. Clarke DE, Vaughan L, Raffin TA. Noninvasive positive pressure ventilation for patients with terminal respiratory failure: the ethical and economic costs of delaying the inevitable are too great. Am J Crit Care 1994;3:4-5.
11. Udwadia ZF, Santis GK, Stevan MH, et al. Nasal ventilation to facilitate weaning in patients with chronic respiratory insufficiency. Thorax 1992;47:715-718.
12. Restrick LJ, Scott AD, Ward EM, et al. Nasal intermittent positive-pressure ventilation in weaning intubated patients with chronic respiratory disease from assisted intermittent positive-pressure ventilation. Respir Med 1993;87:199-204.
13. Nava S, Ambrosino N, Clini E, et al. Noninvasive mechanical ventilation in the weaning of patients with respiratory failure due to chronic obstructive pulmonary disease: a randomized study. Ann Intern Med 1998;128:721-728.
14. Girault C, Daudenthun I, Chevron V, et al. Noninvasive ventilation as a systematic extubation and weaning technique in acute-on-chronic respiratory failure. Am J Resir Crit Care Med 1999;160:86-92.
15. Gregoretti C, Beltrame F, Lucangelo U, et al. Physiologic evaluation of noninvasive pressure support ventilation in trauma patients with acute respiratory failure. Intensive Care Med 1998;24:785-790.
16. Kilger E, Briegel J, Haller M, et al. Effects of noninvasive positive pressure ventilatory support in non-COPD patients with acute respiratory insufficiency after early extubation. Intensive Care Med 1999;25:1374-1380.
17. Hill NS, Lin D, Levy M, et al. Noninvasive positive pressure ventilation (NPPV) to facilitate extubation after acute respiratory failure: a feasibility study. Am J Respir Crit Care Med 2000;161:A263.
18. Epstein SK, Ciabotaru RL, Wong JB. Effect of failed extubation on outcome of mechanical ventilation. Am J Respir Crit Care Med 1997;112:186-192.
19. Goodenberger DM, Couser JI, May JJ. Successful discontinuation of ventilation via tracheostomy by substitution of nasal positive pressure ventilation. Chest 1992;102:1277-1279.
20. Laier-Groeneveld G, Kupfer J, Hutteman U, Criee CP. Weaning from invasive mechanical ventilation. Am Rev Respir Dis 1992;145:A518.
21. Viroslav J, Rosenblatt R, Morris-Tomazevic S. Respiratory management, survival, and quality of life for high-level traumatic tetraplegics. Respir Care Clin North Am 1996;2:313-322.
22. Chevron V, Menard JF, Richard JC, et al. Unplanned extubation: risk factors of development and predictive criteria for reintubation. Crit Care Med 1998;26:1049-1053.
23. Meduri GU, Turner RE, Abou-Shala N, et al. Noninvasive positive pressure ventilation via face mask. Chest 1996;109:179-193.
24. Hilbert G, Gruson D, Gbikpi-Benissan G, Cardinaud JP. Sequential use of noninvasive pressure support ventilation for acute exacerbations of COPD. Intensive Care Med 1997;23:955-961.
25. Jiang J-S, Kao S-J, and Wang S-N. Effect of early application of biphasic positive airway pressure on the outcome of extubation in ventilator weaning. Respirology 1999;4:161-165.

Chapter 7

Nasal Positive Pressure Ventilation in Restrictive Thoracic and Central Hypoventilatory Disorders

Patrick Leger, M.D., Nicholas S. Hill, M.D.

Introduction

Restrictive thoracic disorders cause restrictive pulmonary syndromes and, eventually, chronic alveolar hypoventilation. Untreated, the functional status and life expectancy of patients with restrictive pulmonary syndromes is considerably reduced due to the debilitating effects of respiratory insufficiency. Long-term mechanical ventilation can greatly improve quality of life and survival in these patients, as learned during the polio epidemics of the 1930s through 1950s.[1,2] Initially, negative pressure noninvasive ventilators predominated as the ventilators of choice for patients with chronic respiratory failure due to restrictive thoracic disorders. Since the mid 1980s, however, noninvasive positive pressure ventilation (NPPV) has become the ventilatory mode of first choice for such patients, even over invasive ventilation, as long as patients can cooperate and protect their airway. This chapter will examine the evidence demonstrating that NPPV is the treatment of choice for respiratory insufficiency in restrictive thoracic and central hypoventilatory disorders, discuss principles of patient selection, and provide logical treatment guidelines for these applications.

Definitions

The group of restrictive disorders includes thoracic deformities and neuromuscular diseases. Table 1 lists the main conditions in this group of diseases that may necessitate long-term NPPV. Central hypoventilatory disorders are characterized by a failure of the respiratory center

From *Noninvasive Positive Pressure Ventilation: Principles and Applications,* edited by Nicholas S. Hill. © 2001, Futura Publishing Company, Inc., Armonk, NY.

Table 1

Main Restrictive Thoracic and Central Hyperventilatory
Diseases that May Necessitate Long-Term NPPV

Chest wall deformities
Idiopathic kyphoscoliosis > 100°
Mutilating sequelae of tuberculosis: thoracoplasty, fibrothorax

Neuromuscular disorders
Nonprogressive or slowly progressive (over decades)
Spinal cord injury: tetraplegia (> C5)
Sequelae of poliomyelitis
Diaphragmatic paralysis
Spinal muscular atrophy II and III
Progressive (years to decades)
Congenital myopathies
Metabolic myopathies
Duchenne's muscular dystrophy
Rapidly progressive (months to years)
Amyotrophic lateral sclerosis

Central hypoventilation syndromes
Primary alveolar hypoventilation (Ondine's curse)
Acquired central hypoventilatory disorders
Mixed defects
Obesity hypoventilation syndrome

---

to respond appropriately to chemical stimuli (particularly CO_2), and include congenital primary alveolar hypoventilation (sometimes referred to as Ondine's curse).[3] Central hypoventilation can also be acquired after central vascular insults, central involvement by neoplasms, drug effects, and so on. Some patients, such as those with obesity hypoventilation syndrome, have CO_2 retention resulting from combined defects consisting of blunting of central drive and mechanical defects resulting from the chest wall and abdominal adiposity.

The number of patients with severe chest wall deformities is decreasing as survivors of the polio epidemics and mutilating surgery for tuberculosis (TB) gradually succumb, and new patients with these conditions become rare. This is due to several medical milestones: the development of the polio vaccine during the 1950s, surgical procedures to correct and stabilize spinal deformities during the 1960s, and the effective treatment of TB with antibiotics, eliminating the need for thoracoplasty and pulmonary resection to treat this disease. On the other hand, use of NPPV in patients with congenital myopathies and amyotrophic lateral sclerosis (motor neuron disease) is increasing as the technology improves and more clinicians become familiar with its application.

Natural History

For restrictive disorders, respiratory dysfunction is typically slowly progressive. Patients tolerate their disability without major respiratory complaints for long periods of time and usually have active lives. This is especially true for patients with chest wall deformities who may not seek medical treatment until 40 or 50 years of age. For neuromuscular patients, symptoms of hypoventilation appear at various ages according to the disease.[4] Severe disability, cardiac failure, and eventual death follow untreated, progressive deterioration in respiratory status. Neuromuscular diseases can be classified according to their potential progressiveness as seen in Table 1. These distinctions are important, because patients with stable or slowly progressive disease can adapt themselves well to their handicap, even when it is very severe. On the other hand, rapidly progressive diseases like amyotrophic lateral sclerosis (ALS) are much more difficult for patients and families to cope with because of their relentless progression. Further, ALS tends to strike middle-aged or older individuals who may be less adaptable than their younger counterparts with muscular dystrophies.

Clinical Concerns

In general, restrictive patients should have their pulmonary functions and symptoms monitored on a yearly basis and more often when their vital capacities drop below 50% of predicted value or < 1.5 L, and when respiratory muscle strength as measured by the maximal inspiratory force drops below 50% of predicted value.[5] Common medical concerns for restrictive patients include respiratory muscle weakness, sleep-disordered breathing, cor pulmonale, and oxygen desaturation during exercise (Table 2). Additional concerns specific to patients with neuromuscular disease include physical limitations related to muscular weakness, cardiac involvement in some myopathies, severe expiratory muscle weakness leading to impairment of the ability to cough, and upper airway dysfunction interfering with the swallowing mechanism. Associated risk factors such as obesity, pregnancy, smoking, obstructive lung disease, or bronchiectasis (frequently seen in patients with old TB)

Table 2
Common Medical Concerns in Restrictive Disorders

	Thoracic Deformity	Neuromuscular Diseases
Inspiratory muscle weakness	+	++
Expiratory muscle weakness	+	+++
Impaired cough		+++
Sleep-disordered breathing	++	++
Cor pulmonale	+	±
Cardiomyopathy		+
Upper airway dysfunction		++
Exercise desaturation	+	±

+, occasional; ++, common; +++, very common; ±, not common but may occur.

significantly aggravate the respiratory impairment in these patients. Respiratory tract infections and surgery also commonly precipitate medical crises in restrictive patients.

Symptoms and signs that should signal the need for a prompt and in-depth evaluation include worsening dyspnea or orthopnea, a decrease in the ability to perform the activities of daily living, and signs of cor pulmonale. The earliest manifestation of dysfunction usually occurs during rapid eye movement (REM) sleep, when the normal hypotonia of upper airway and chest wall muscles is enhanced, leading to increased upper airway resistance and hypoventilation.[6] Deterioration in nocturnal gas exchange causes arousals and poor quality of sleep, leading to symptoms of nocturnal or morning headaches, daytime fatigue and hypersomnolence, decreased intellectual performance, irritability and, occasionally, enuresis. In addition, symptoms may occur insidiously, manifesting themselves as loss of appetite and weight, an increase in the number of calls for assistance during the night, the inability to lay flat during physical therapy, or restless sleep. Such symptoms should raise the suspicion of a deteriorating respiratory status, and clinicians should never merely prescribe hypnotics to such patients without first evaluating gas exchange. Otherwise a respiratory crisis could be precipitated by a well-intentioned benzodiazepine prescription.

Efficacy of NPPV in Restrictive Thoracic Disorders

Goals

When patients with restrictive thoracic disorders develop respiratory insufficiency, goals of ventilatory assistance should be to maintain stability of gas exchange, optimize comfort with the ventilator, minimize symptoms, eliminate signs of cor pulmonale, improve the patient's quality of life, reduce morbidity, and extend survival, all achieved in a cost-effective manner (Table 3). These goals can be realized only by institution of a comprehensive treatment plan that includes rehabilitation to optimize the patient's level of functioning. Such a program should include physical and occupational therapy evaluations as well as the teaching of assisted cough maneuvers to caregivers. Adequate oxygenation is another goal of noninvasive ventilation, although long-term oxygen therapy (LTOT) is rarely needed once adequate ventilatory assistance has been established, unless the patient has underlying parenchymal lung disease. In fact, LTOT alone is poorly tolerated in stable hypercapnic neuromuscular patients; it induces a significant further rise in $PaCO_2$, and should thus be avoided.[7]

Early Responses

The efficacy of noninvasive ventilation in restrictive thoracic disorders can be discussed in terms of early and long-term results. Table 4 summarizes results of studies showing the main clinical responses that can be expected with the use of NPPV in restrictive disorders.

Symptoms

Patients often experience alleviation of their symptoms within the first few nights to weeks of NPPV therapy. Morning headaches and daytime hypersomnolence are usually the first to respond. Such a re-

---

Table 3
Goals of Long-Term Noninvasive
Ventilation in Restrictive Thoracic Disorders

- Improve and stabilize gas exchange
- Ameliorate symptoms
- Eliminate cor pulmonale
- Improve sleep quality
- Improve quality of life
- Optimize comfort during ventilation
- Minimize risk and morbidity
- Extend survival
- Cost-effective management

Table 4
Main Clinical Responses Obtained with Nocturnal NPPV*

Variable	Clinical Responses			
Initial PaO$_2$ and change after 1 year of NPPV (PaO$_2$ and change are in mm Hg)	Scoliosis	54	+10	(8)
	Sequelae of TB	52	+ 8	(8)
	Duchenne's dystrophy	75	+12	(8)
	Neuromuscular	56	+14	(9)
		56	+20	(6)
Initial PaCO$_2$ and change after 1 year of NPPV (PaCO$_2$ and change are in mm Hg)	Scoliosis	53	−10	(8)
	Sequelae of TB	54	− 7	(8)
	Duchenne's dystrophy	52	− 8	(8)
	Neuromuscular	61	−11	(9)
		62	−15	(6)
Sleep				
Subjective	Improved (8,10)			
Total sleep time	Improved (10,11)			
Efficiency	Improved (10,11)			
Nocturnal oxygenation	Improved (6)			
Pulmonary function tests	Unchanged (6)			
Inspiratory muscle force	Improved (6)			
Inspiratory muscle endurance	Improved (11)			
Quality of life	Scoliosis, sequelae of TB: improved (11) Neuromuscular: improved (12,13)			
Noncompliance (% of patients who voluntarily interrupt NPPV)	Scoliosis	7% (8)	0% (9)	
	Sequelae of TB	1% (8)	0% (9)	
	Neuromuscular	0% (8)		
Reduction in the number of days of hospitalization comparing before and after initiation of NPPV	Significant for all restrictive patients during the first 2 years (8)			

*Number in parenthesis indicates reference number.

sponse is propitious because the positive feeling reinforces continued use of the therapy.

Gas Exchange

Normalization of arterial blood gases is usually obtainable during ventilation in restrictive patients, at least in patients with neuromuscular disease who usually have no parenchymal lung disease per se. Prevention of nocturnal hypoventilation also has major effects on gas exchange while awake. Normalization of the $PaCO_2$ during sleep is thought to enhance central chemoreceptor sensitivity, which may have become blunted during the gradual development of hypercapnic respiratory failure.[14] The resetting of the respiratory center is one of the main theories, along with improved respiratory muscle strength, to explain the improvement in daytime spontaneous ventilation associated with nocturnal ventilatory assistance.[15] This occurs over a period of days and/or weeks, with a gradual reduction in daytime $PaCO_2$. Once a plateau is reached, daytime $PaCO_2$s tend to remain stable for long periods of time, depending on the natural history of the underlying disorder.[16] This improvement in gas exchange is usually significant enough to allow patients to be completely free from supplemental oxygen or ventilation during the day and, for most, during exercise.

Sleep

Early on, patients report an improved quality of sleep after initiating nocturnal NPPV. This response may not be immediate, because patients usually require some time (days to weeks) to successfully adapt. However, sleep quality is almost invariably improved by nocturnal NPPV at some point, both objectively, as evidenced by increases in total sleep time and sleep efficiency, and subjectively, as patients notice less daytime sleepiness and an improved sense of well being.[6,17]

Long-Term Responses

Gas Exchange

As shown in Table 4, different studies report similar results with regard to improvements in daytime PaO_2 and $PaCO_2$ levels. These blood gases were obtained during spontaneous breathing, several hours after ventilation. The values remain remarkably steady during the day in between sessions of nocturnal ventilation.[16] In patients with thoracovertebral deformities, the improvement is usually 10–15 mm Hg for both PaO_2 and $PaCO_2$ during spontaneous breathing. Complete normalization of daytime $PaCO_2$ may be difficult to achieve in these patients, because of the severity of the mechanical ventilatory defect. Once achieved, though, this improvement persists indefinitely,[8] because of the relative stability of the underlying defect.

In patients with progressive neuromuscular diseases, on the other hand, additional hours of ventilation during the day may be necessary to maintain stability of gas exchange. The need for increasing periods of ventilation is determined by the rate of disease progression, and the rate of increase in daytime $PaCO_2$. The ideal level of daytime $PaCO_2$ for patients with restrictive thoracic diseases receiving long-term NPPV is a matter of debate. Some investigators recommend normalizing the daytime $PaCO_2$,[18] but others advocate accepting a level above normal (up to 50–60 mm Hg) as long as the patient's symptoms of hypoventilation and signs of cor pulmonale are controlled.[15] The latter strategy allows patients to maintain a steady level of gas exchange at a lower minute volume than would be necessary to normalize $PaCO_2$.

Pulmonary Function

There has long been a debate about whether or not long-term NPPV acts by improving respiratory muscle function. One theory has held that NPPV works in patients with chronic respiratory failure by resting chronically fatigued respiratory muscles, thereby improving pulmonary function.[19] The improved pulmonary function would translate into better gas exchange and, ultimately, improved overall function. However, reported changes in pulmonary function and respiratory muscle force have been inconsistent.[16,20] Some studies have observed increases in vital capacity and maximal inspiratory and expiratory pressures after periods of noninvasive ventilation,[21,22] but these were uncontrolled, and could not exclude the possibility that improvements in gas exchange alone were responsible for the improved pulmonary function.[23] Some studies have detected improvements in more subtle indices of respiratory muscle function, such as the maximum sustained breathing capacity.[11] However, others have observed stability in gas exchange despite steadily declining pulmonary function (in progressive muscular dystrophies),[16] demonstrating that the benefits of NPPV do not rely on improvements in pulmonary function.

Survival

The life expectancy of restrictive patients not treated for respiratory failure is significantly reduced.[24,25] Duchenne's muscular dystrophy patients die of respiratory failure at an average age of 20 years.[4] Fifty percent of ALS patients die 3 years after the diagnosis, and only 10% are alive at 10 years.[26] For scoliotic patients who develop chronic hypoventilation complicated by cor pulmonale, 50% die within the first year and 80% after 2 years.[27] Long-term oxygen therapy alone may improve the prognosis in some patients with chronic respiratory failure,[27,28] but it has already been emphasized that such an approach in hypercapnic patients with neuromuscular disease may promote greater CO_2 retention.[7]

Although no randomized controlled trials have been performed, there can be little question that NPPV prolongs survival in patients with restrictive thoracic disorders. Table 5 lists the results of different studies concerning long-term home respiratory assistance in patients with kyphoscoliosis and sequelae of TB. Results are reported as survival or the probability to continue therapy using Kaplan-Meier analysis. As can be seen in the table, Robert et al.[28] reported in 1983 that the use of tracheostomy positive pressure ventilation (TPPV) was associated with a remarkably high survival rate in patients with chest wall deformities after 5 years of treatment. Two other studies[8,9] showed similar results in comparable but larger populations of restrictive patients treated with NPPV. Comparing these studies of similar patients shows that when patients use either invasive or noninvasive ventilation, their likelihood of continuing therapy at 5 years is much better than surviving with oxygen therapy alone.[29]

Table 5
Survival or the Probability to Continue Long-Term Home Respiratory Assistance for Patients with Kyphoscoliosis or Tuberculosis

| | Reference | Number of Patients | Patient Survival or Contraindication of NPPV Years* | | | | |
			1	2	3	4	5
KS LTOT	Robert[28]	27	88	83	60	60	60
KS NPPV	Leger[8]	105	90	80	78	76	73
KS NPPV	Simond[9]	47	90	90	79	79	79
KS TPPV	Robert[29]	53	88	88	86	86	77
TB LTOT	Robert[28]	70	78	65	56	53	53
TB NPPV	Leger[8]	80	86	79	75	67	60
TB NPPV	Simond[9]	20	94	94	94	94	94
TB TPPV	Robert[29]	55	100	94	81	73	70

*Numbers are percentages.
KS, idiopathic kyphoscoliosis; TB, mutilating sequelae of tuberculosis; LTOT, probability of survival on long-term oxygen therapy; NPPV, probability of continuing nasal positive pressure ventilation; TPPV, probability of survival on tracheostomy positive pressure ventilation.

Outcomes of long-term studies of NPPV in neuromuscular diseases are quite varied, and once again, there are no randomized controlled trials. Vianello et al.[30] observed the survival outcomes of 10 patients with Duchenne's muscular dystrophy. All 5 patients who used NPPV survived the next 2 years, whereas 4 of 5 who declined assisted ventilation died. For patients with sequelae of poliomyelitis (an almost nonprogressive disease) studied by Simonds and Elliott,[9] the continuation rate after 5 years was 100%. For various other neuromuscular patients, the 5-year probability to continue NPPV was 81%. In the French study,[8] Duchenne's muscular dystrophy was the only neuromuscular disease studied. Results were less successful than in the Simonds and Elliott study, with a probability to continue NPPV of 47%. The majority of patients who failed to continue NPPV were switched to TPPV and were still alive. Duchenne's muscular dystrophy patients who continue NPPV extend the duration of ventilation to 24 hours as their disease progresses, often using mouthpiece ventilation during the day.[31]

Survival has also been examined in ALS, one of the most challenging of the restrictive disorders because of its rapid progression and proclivity to bulbar involvement. In a retrospective analysis, Gay et al.[32] reported success in 7 of 9 patients with ALS as part of a larger series of patients using nasal ventilation. These 7 patients had improvements in gas exchange and symptoms, and 1 patient remained stable after 26 months. However, 3 of the 7 died within 6 months, and most of the survivors had been ventilated for only a year or less. In a nonrandomized prospective trial, Pinto et al.[26] used nasal BiPAP in 10 ALS patients with an average vital capacity of 48% of the predicted value. The control group had an average vital capacity of 64% of predicted value and received regular medical treatment without ventilation. During the follow-up period, all controls died within 8 months, whereas the group using BiPAP had a 55% survival at 24 months. More recently, Aboussouan et al.[33] found that nasal NPPV was tolerated in 18 of 39 (46%) patients with respiratory insufficiency due to ALS. Risk of death was reduced by a factor of 3.1 if the patient tolerated NPPV. Risk of death was also reduced in patients with bulbar involvement who tolerated NPPV, even though swallowing dysfunction is ordinarily considered a relative contraindication to the use of noninvasive ventilation. Bulbar involvement halved the likelihood of tolerating the device, however.

Even with the lack of controls, these studies demonstrate beyond a reasonable doubt that NPPV extends survival in patients with restrictive thoracic disorders, but outcomes are highly dependent on the natural history of the underlying process. For instance, survival is much better in relatively static conditions like severe chest wall deformity or poliomyelitis, and much worse for rapidly progressive neuromuscular conditions like Duchenne's muscular dystrophy or ALS. Because the uncontrolled trials are so favorable, it is unlikely that randomized controlled trials will ever be performed to prove that NPPV extends survival in patients with restrictive thoracic disorders. The efficacy of this approach seems so clear that most investigators would consider it unethical to perform such a randomized trial.

Quality of Life, Need for Hospitalization, and Compliance with Therapy

The quality of life with NPPV has been evaluated using questionnaires.[12,13,34] Patients with restrictive disorders using NPPV consistently have improvements in chronic hypoventilation symptoms, and a better quality of sleep. In a survey by Simonds,[34] 73% of the patients said that they were less tired, 44% said they were less breathless, and 48% reported a decreased frequency of respiratory infections. The majority of patients were able to return to work at home and some returned to professional work. In addition, these patients were hospitalized less frequently. A comparison of the year before and after initiation of nasal ventilation from the French study[8] revealed a decrease in the number of hospital days from 34 days to 5 days for scoliosis patients and from 31 days to 9 days for patients with sequelae of TB (both p<0.05). This emphasizes the stability of most patients and the fact that hospitalizations for acute exacerbations are often averted once NPPV is begun. Compliance with therapy was also generally very high despite the constraints imposed by the mask and ventilator; 7% of scoliosis patients, 1% of the patients with sequelae of TB, and 0% of Duchenne's muscular dystrophy patients discontinued ventilation during the course of the study (Table 4).[8] In the Simonds and Elliott study,[9] mean NPPV use was 7.88 hours per 24 hours for 43 monitored patients, as determined by a clock hidden in the ventilator. Compliance with therapy appears to be related to the degree of improvement as perceived by the patient.

Effects of Temporary Cessation of NPPV

Considering that a randomized, prospective trial designed to determine whether NPPV improves survival would be considered unethical, several groups of investigators have temporarily withdrawn NPPV from patients with restrictive thoracic disorders.[15,35] In these studies, patients had presented with symptoms and arterial blood gases compatible with chronic alveolar hypoventilation, which had responded favorably to NPPV. The authors hypothesized that if NPPV was effective, then temporary withdrawal would lead to a decline in clinical status. In all of the studies, patients deteriorated during the period of withdrawal. The earliest and most dramatic change was the reappearance of nocturnal hypoventilation during the period without any assisted ventilation, especially during REM sleep.[15,35] Sleep quality also deteriorated[35] with a marked increase in the frequency of arousals. Symptoms of fatigue, morning headache, and daytime hypersomnolence recurred soon thereafter. Interestingly, measures of pulmonary function did not change significantly during the period of withdrawal.[15] After resumption of NPPV, nocturnal hypoventilation and symptoms once again resolved, and sleep quality was restored.

These studies demonstrate that NPPV is effective at controlling nocturnal hypoventilation and symptoms in patients with chronic respiratory failure due to restrictive thoracic diseases. They are also compatible with the idea that NPPV works in these patients by preventing nocturnal hypoventilation and restoring respiratory center sensitivity to CO_2, thereby lowering daytime CO_2.[15] Further evidence to support the idea that NPPV improves gas exchange by enhancing respiratory center responsiveness to CO_2 derives from a study by Annane et al.,[36] showing an increase in the slope of the ventilatory response curve to CO_2 that was sustained for at least 3 years after patients began NPPV, in the absence of any change in vital capacity.

Schonhofer et al.[37] have demonstrated that noninvasive ventilatory assistance need not be nocturnal to lower $PaCO_2$. These investigators ventilated 34 hypercapnic patients for 8 hours per 24 hours either nocturnally, or during the daytime. Patients receiving daytime ventilation were kept awake during ventilation periods by using a signal generator. The reduction in $PaCO_2$ was equivalent whether patients were ventilated during the daytime or nocturnally. Although these investigators did not monitor daytime sleep, their findings suggest that, as long as patients receive ventilatory assistance for at least a portion of the time (probable minimum 4–6 hr/24 hr), the respiratory center sensitivity to CO_2 will be reset regardless of the sleep state. This also indicated that patients unable to sleep during ventilator use will still derive benefit even if they use NPPV only during the daytime.

Evidence for Efficacy of NPPV in Central Hypoventilatory Disorders or Obstructive Sleep Apnea

The first case reports describing the use of nasal ventilation for chronic respiratory failure were in young children with central hypoventilation.[38,39] These patients had resolution of gas exchange abnormalities and symptoms after initiation of therapy. Subsequently, little additional information has accrued on this application and there have been no controlled studies. However, there is enough anecdotal evidence so that consensus groups now consider therapy of central hypoventilation as an appropriate indication for NPPV.[40] These patients usually come to clinical attention because of symptoms of chronic hypoventilation and manifest CO_2 retention at the time of their initial visit. Accordingly, they are promptly started on NPPV, and because their lungs and upper airway function are otherwise intact, they generally respond well to therapy.

With regard to obstructive sleep apnea, nasal CPAP is considered the therapy of first choice. However, when patients with severe obstructive sleep apnea present with frank respiratory failure and fail to respond to continuous positive airway pressure (CPAP), NPPV may be necessary to improve daytime gas exchange and symptoms.[41] These patients are often morbidly obese, and "bilevel" ventilators may not successfully ventilate them because of the high airway pressures necessary. Portable volume-limited ventilators are suitable alternatives for these patents. Bilevel ventilation has been touted in patients with obstructive sleep apnea as a way to reduce discomfort and improve compliance by virtue of the reduction in positive pressure during expiration.[42] However, Reeves-Hoche et al.[43] were unable to demonstrate improved compliance rates in patients with obstructive sleep apnea treated with bilevel ventilation compared to CPAP alone. Hence, use of NPPV for obstructive apnea should be reserved for those patients who have persisting hypoventilation despite adequate CPAP therapy.

Few studies have examined the efficacy of NPPV in obesity-hypoventilation syndrome. Pankow et al.[44] demonstrated a 40% reduction in inspiratory muscle activity among 18 patients with a body mass index $> 40 \text{ kg/m}^2$ when treated with bilevel ventilation. In a preliminary report, Muir et al.[45] successfully treated 18 of 20 morbidly obese acute respiratory failure patients with noninvasive ventilation using either pressure or volume-limited ventilators. They found more rapid improvement in gas exchange using pressure-limited ventilation and suggested that bilevel ventilation should be used as first-line therapy. These reports show promise for this application of NPPV, but lacking controlled studies, only tentative recommendations can be made regarding specific indications or the preferred techniques.

Criteria for the Initiation of NPPV in Restrictive Patients

Based on the accumulated evidence regarding efficacy described above, criteria have been proposed in a recent consensus document for the initiation of NPPV in restrictive patients.[46] As listed in Table 6, the presence of symptoms of hypoventilation signals the need for further evaluation with arterial blood gases. Arterial blood gases for restrictive patients that warrant initiation of NPPV include a daytime/awake $PaCO_2 > 45$ mm Hg. In addition, a decline in vital capacity to $< 50\%$ predicted may be considered an indication for initiation when combined with symptoms, particularly in patients with rapidly progressive neuromuscular processes such as ALS.

For symptomatic patients without daytime blood gas abnormalities, nocturnal monitoring of gas exchange is indicated. Nocturnal monitoring includes continuous SpO_2 and arterial blood gases early in the morning to detect nocturnal hypoventilation. End-tidal or transcutaneous CO_2 monitoring may be useful, but results of these are not sufficiently accurate to entirely replace blood gases.[47] NPPV is indicated if O_2 saturation remains $< 88\%$ for more than 5 consecutive minutes, consistent with sustained nocturnal hypoventilation, even in the absence of daytime hypoventilation. If daytime hypoventilation is absent, airflow at the nose and chest wall motion should also be monitored to detect evidence of obstructive sleep apnea, which could respond to CPAP alone.

Table 6
Criteria for Initiation of NPPV in Restrictive Patients*

Clinical symptoms or signs of hypoventilation:
1. Daytime ventilation: $PaCO_2 > 45$, or
2. Sustained nocturnal desaturation (O_2 sat $\leq 88\%$ for > 5 consecutive minutes on usual FiO_2), or
3. Severe ventilatory restriction (FVC $< 50\%$ predicted) wth a rapidly progressive process, or
4. After repeated hospitalizations in setting of severe restriction.

*Adapted from reference 46.

Another indication for initiation of long-term noninvasive ventilation in patients with severe restrictive thoracic disorders is repeated admissions for acute respiratory failure. There are often life-threatening events that can usually be managed with ventilatory assistance and aggressive pulmonary toilet. Because respiratory infections complicated by acute secretion retention usually precipitate these crises, initial intubation is often necessary, and the patient is eventually weaned to noninvasive ventilation. Because of the high probability of recurrent hospitalizations for bouts of respiratory failure, long-term noninvasive ventilation should be considered. The same gas exchange and clinical criteria listed in Table 6 can be used after an acute exacerbation to decide on the need for continued NPPV.

How Early to Start Noninvasive Ventilation in Restrictive Patients

The issue of when to start NPPV in patients with restrictive thoracic disorders has garnered debate. Some clinicians believe that early initiation of NPPV in patients with progressive neuromuscular disorders slows the rate of pulmonary function deterioration.[48] To test this hypothesis, Raphael et al.[49] randomized patients with Duchenne's muscular dystrophy to receive NPPV or conventional therapy before they developed symptoms or CO_2 retention. After a mean follow-up period of 52 months, 10 of 35 (28%) patients in the NPPV arm had died as compared with only 2 of 35 (6%) patients in the conventional therapy arm ($p < 0.05$). Further, there was no indication of a slowing in the decline of pulmonary function. With the greater mortality in the NPPV arm, the trial was stopped. The study has been criticized for failing to monitor patient compliance with NPPV and for inclusion in the NPPV group of more patients with left ventricular hypokinesis than among controls. Thus, firm conclusions about the effect of NPPV on mortality cannot be made. Nevertheless, these findings suggest that "prophylactic" use of NPPV in Duchenne's muscular dystrophy patients is not useful in retarding progression of the underlying process.

On the other hand, available evidence suggests that clinicians need not wait for daytime hypoventilation in restrictive thoracic disorders before starting NPPV. Masa et al.[50] identified 27 patients with restrictive thoracic disorders who were symptomatic with sustained nocturnal oxygen desaturations (<90% for an average of 39% of sleep time) but without daytime hypercapnia. After initiation of NPPV, symptoms and nocturnal desaturations resolved. The authors concluded that initiation of NPPV in symptomatic patients with significant nocturnal desaturations, even before the onset of daytime CO_2 retention, is warranted to prevent the development of respiratory failure.

Thus, based on current knowledge, NPPV should be started in patients with neuromuscular disease when they develop symptoms of hypoventilation, such as excessive fatigue, daytime hypersomnolence, and morning headache. Most clinicians believe that patients who start NPPV before the onset of at least some symptoms are unlikely to comply with the therapy. However, some patients deny symptoms or are unaware of them until treatment brings alleviation, so NPPV may be started in those with severe pulmonary dysfunction if a sleep study shows sustained desaturations, or substantial daytime CO_2 retention has occurred (i.e., $PaCO_2 > 50$ mm Hg).

With the onset of symptoms, pulmonary functions, nocturnal oximetry and a daytime arterial blood gas should also be obtained. If sustained nocturnal desaturations or significant hypercarbia are found, NPPV should be started. An important point is that the onset of respiratory deterioration in patients with neuromuscular disease can be subtle, and the astute clinician will monitor pulmonary functions periodically and warn patients to report the insidious onset of symptoms. If NPPV is started at the first sign of clinical deterioration, even before the onset of daytime hypoventilation, respiratory crises can often be averted.

Application of Noninvasive Ventilation to Restrictive Patients

When a patient with a restrictive thoracic disorder presents with symptomatic chronic respiratory failure, NPPV is the initial method of choice. Patients with neuromuscular disease and acute respiratory failure, on the other hand, often have difficulty expectorating secretions and may require initial intubation. Once stabilized, however, these patients should then be weaned to NPPV, if possible. As discussed in Chapter 1, volume- or pressure-limited devices or bilevel units can be used; the choice is largely determined by practitioner and patient preferences, efficacy in controlling nocturnal hypoventilation, and the level of ventilator dependency.

For restrictive patients in need of nocturnal ventilation alone, portable bilevel (or pressure support) devices are a good first choice. These synchronize well with patient breathing efforts, or can be set with a sufficiently high backup rate to control the patient's breathing during sleep, something many neuromuscular patients seem to prefer. Suggested initial inspiratory and expiratory pressure settings are 8–10 cm H_2O and 3–4 cm H_2O, respectively. The former is gradually titrated upward as tolerated by the patient (to 12–20 cm H_2O) until the targeted daytime $PaCO_2$ level is reached. The expiratory positive airway pressure is usually kept at some minimum level to control rebreathing (3–4 cm H_2O), depending on the device and valve system. Higher positive end-expiratory pressure (PEEP) levels may be necessary, however, to maintain airway patency in patients with underlying obstructive sleep apnea or to improve oxygenation in patients with underlying parenchymal lung disease. The ideal target for a daytime $PaCO_2$ has not been established, although levels in the 40s mm Hg are desirable. In the authors' experience, however, levels in the 60s may be well tolerated as long as symptoms and evidence of cor pulmonale are controlled. This approach permits very debilitated patients to breathe free of the ventilator for periods during the daytime because a lower minute volume is required than that necessary to maintain a lower $PaCO_2$.

Patients with a high level of ventilator dependency are often provided with portable volume-limited ventilators because of enhanced alarm and monitoring capabilities compared with bilevel ventilators, the availability of internal and external batteries, the ability to "stack" breaths (see below), and amenability for mounting on a wheelchair. If a volume-limited ventilator is chosen, restrictive patients tend to prefer a set frequency close to their spontaneous breathing frequency and a relatively high tidal volume, around 10–15 mL/kg. However, these distinctions between pressure- and volume-limited ventilators are becoming blurred as newer microprocessor ventilators are being introduced that are capable of delivering both pressure- and volume-limited modes of ventilation, have sophisticated alarm and monitoring capabilities, and are sufficiently compact to be used in the home or mounted on a wheelchair (see Chapter 1). In fact, one of these, the Pulmonetics LTV 1000 (Colton, CA) is no larger than a laptop computer and weighs only 5.8 kg.

With the exception of patients with underlying parenchymal lung disease or acute respiratory failure, supplemental O_2 is usually unnecessary in restrictive patients. Thus, ventilator settings are best initiated on room air. In fact, supplemental O_2 may obscure changes in ventilation as detected by changes in oxygen saturation. Titration on room air allows the clinician to focus on decreasing the CO_2, which is the most effective way to relieve symptoms. After the initial adjustments, subsequent settings and the duration of ventilation are adjusted according to the arterial blood gases and the ability to reduce daytime

$PaCO_2$. Patients with acute respiratory failure may initially need 24-hour ventilation to obtain targeted blood gas values. The duration of ventilation may then be decreased as the patient recovers from the initial problem. This may take several weeks to several months.

In patients with chronic respiratory failure, the opposite approach is taken, with patients using the ventilator as tolerated initially, sometimes amounting to as little as 1 or 2 hours per day. Ventilator periods are then gradually increased over a period of weeks to months until gas exchange targets are reached and other goals are met.

As discussed in Chapter 2, successful initiation of noninvasive ventilation depends on proper interface selection and fitting. Specific interface concerns related to restrictive patients include ease of attachment and removal, considering that many patients have limited upper extremity function. Oral leaks are frequent in restrictive patients, particularly in those with bulbar involvement. In this situation, mouthpiece or full face mask ventilation at night should be considered, but there is an asphyxiation risk should the ventilator malfunction in a patient unable to remove the mask. Some manufacturers have installed "anti-asphyxia" valves in their full face masks to address this problem. Alternatively, a SONI (strapless oral nasal interface) should be considered for patients who have significant mouth leaks and upper extremity weakness.[18] For patients unable to maintain desired daytime arterial blood gas levels with nocturnal ventilation alone, daytime ventilation should be added. For patients using wheelchairs, this can easily be accomplished by using a simple angled mouthpiece suspended from a gooseneck clamp. Patients should be counseled on how to incorporate daytime ventilation into their normal daily activities. Many hours of ventilation can be accumulated during the day with intermittent use.

When initiating NPPV in patients with advanced neuromuscular disease, attention should be paid not only to ventilatory limitations, but also to cough impairment. Because of expiratory muscle weakness and limited inspiratory capacity, these patients are unable to generate the expiratory flows necessary to cough effectively, especially during respiratory infections.[51] Accordingly, patients should have their ability to cough checked during follow-up visits. If cough is determined to be weakened, caregivers should be instructed in manually assisted ("quad") coughing techniques. Patients with severe cough impairment should also be considered for mechanical aids to coughing such as percussive devices or the cough In-Exsufflator (JH Emerson, Cambridge, MA) (see Chapter 1).[51] The cough In-Exsufflator uses a positive pressure of 30–40 cm H_2O via a face mask to fully inflate the lungs, and then rapidly switches to an equal negative force to simulate a cough maneuver. Although no controlled trials have been performed on this device to confirm its clinical utility, it has gained popularity in recent years because of anecdotal evdidence suggesting that it can be used to help patients manage respiratory exacerbations in the home.[52]

Contraindications to NPPV in Restrictive Patients

As can be seen in Table 7, contraindications to NPPV are relatively few. The inability to fit or tolerate a mask is the only absolute contraindication. The others are relative and require clinical judgment. The ability to protect the airway is a major concern during noninvasive ventilation because, unlike invasive ventilation, there is no direct access to the lower airways. Thus, patients with severe bulbar involvement, weakness of expiratory muscles, or secretion retention should consider invasive ventilation. On the other hand, the available evidence suggests that even patients with severe bulbar involvement survive longer with noninvasive ventilation than with no ventilatory assistance at all.[33] Thus, if patients with airway compromise decline invasive ventilation, noninvasive ventilation may still be tried. Other relative contraindications include an inability to cooperate or lack of motivation. These may not be clear until the patient has tried to initiate NPPV. It should be borne in mind that because complications of noninvasive ventilation are generally minor, a trial is usually indicated unless it is quite clear that the attempt will be futile.

When to Switch from NPPV to Tracheostomy Ventilation

This is a topic that arouses considerable debate. It is quite clear that patients require a tracheostomy after they have failed a reasonable

---

Table 7
Contraindications to NPPV

Absolute
　Inability to fit or tolerate mask
Relative
　Severe bulbar involvement and swallowing dysfunction
　Lack of patient/family motivation and/or cooperation
　Inability to clear secretions (despite assisted coughing maneuvers)
　Need for continuous ventilatory support

trial of noninvasive ventilation including consideration of alternative noninvasive devices. Also, patients who have required repeated acute intubations despite optimal noninvasive management should undergo tracheostomy. However, the decision is more difficult when determining how much swallowing dysfunction or difficulty clearing secretions warrants a tracheostomy. The arguments for performing tracheostomy in patients with upper airway dysfunction usually center around security issues and facilitation of secretion removal. Those who argue in favor of NPPV point out that patient security is the same or better with NPPV, and that secretion production and problems with airway infection are less with NPPV than with tracheostomy ventilation because of the absence of an irritating tube that bypasses the normal airway defense system. However, if secretion retention is a bothersome problem causing repeated acute episodes of plugging, and the patient wants to maximize survival, a tracheostomy is a sensible option. On the other hand, patients who abhor the need for repeated suctioning and other unsavory aspects of having a tracheostomy will opt to continue with NPPV as long as possible.

Another debatable issue is whether the 24-hour ventilator-dependent patient is better or more safely ventilated by TPPV or NPPV. Some authors have suggested that patients requiring more than 16 hours of assisted ventilation per day should undergo tracheostomy.[53] On the other hand, there are numerous examples of patients having been managed with noninvasive ventilation for 24 hours per day, sometimes for years.[18] In the absence of scientific data relating to this topic, the outcome of the debate for an individual patient will depend mainly on the desires and capabilities of the patient and family as well as the treating team of caregivers.

Conclusions

Despite the growing popularity of evidence-based medicine, the use of noninvasive ventilation for patients with chronic respiratory failure due to restrictive thoracic disorders is an example of a clinical practice becoming established in the absence of randomized controlled trials proving efficacy. The consistently favorable findings of retrospective studies with the additional weight of withdrawal trials has strongly supported the use of mechanical ventilation as the treatment of choice when respiratory insufficiency occurs in patients with restrictive thoracic disorders. Ultimately, though, it has been the consistently favorable clinical responses of individual patients that have convinced clinicians that NPPV is a highly effective therapy for this group of patients. Just as there should never be a randomized placebo-controlled trial of antibiotics for bacterial pneumonia, there should never be a long-term randomized trial of NPPV use in restrictive thoracic patients that includes nonventilated controls.

The approach to providing NPPV to restrictive patients consists of monitoring pulmonary function and symptoms. When pulmonary function becomes marginal or signs and symptoms of respiratory insufficiency develop, further evaluation is warranted to document the onset of nocturnal hypoventilation, preferably before frank respiratory failure has developed. Noninvasive ventilation should be initiated without hesitation in these patients, paying attention to the goals of long-term mechanical ventilation, including amelioration of gas exchange abnormalities and symptoms, improvement in function and in the quality of life, and extension of survival. Patients should be initiated with the unique characteristics of restrictive patients kept in mind, including the tendency for large air leaks through the mouth if bulbar muscles are weakened, and cough impairment in neuromuscular patients. With proper selection of patients and skilled management by an experienced team of clinicians, the vast majority of these patients should be managed successfully with noninvasive ventilation, often for many years.

References

1. Wilson JL. Acute anterior poliomyelitis. N Engl J Med 1932;206:887-893.
2. Plum F, Whedon GD. The rapid-rocking bed: its effect on the ventilation of poliomyelitis patients with respiratory paralysis. N Engl J Med 1951;245:235-240.
3. Reichel J. Primary alveolar hypoventilation. Clin Chest Med 1980;1:119-124.
4. Rideau Y, Jankowski LW, Grellet IJ. Respiratory function in the muscular dystrophies. Muscle Nerve 1981;4:155-164.
5. Braun NMT, Arora NS, Rochester DF. Respiratory muscle and pulmonary function in polymyositis and other proximal myopathies. Thorax 1983;38:616-623.
6. Piper AJ, Sullivan CE. Effects of long-term nocturnal nasal ventilation on spontaneous breathing during sleep in neuromuscular and chest wall disorders. Eur Respir J 1996;9:1515-1522.
7. Gay PC, Edmonds LC. Severe hypercapnia after low-flow oxygen therapy in patients with neuromuscular disease and diaphragmatic dysfunction. Mayo Clin Proc 1995;70(4):327-330.
8. Leger P, Bedicam JM, Cornette A, et al. Nasal IPPV: long term follow up in patients with severe respiratory insufficiency. Chest 1994;105:100-105.

9. Simonds AK, Elliott MW. Outcome of domiciliary nasal positive pressure ventilation in restrictive and obstructive disorders. Thorax 1995;50:604-609.

10. Ellis RE, Bye PT, Bruderer JW, Sullivan CE. Treatment of respiratory failure during sleep in patients with neuromuscular diseases: positive pressure ventilation through a nose mask. Am Rev Respir Dis 1987;135:148-152.

11. Goldstein RS, De Rosle JA, Avendano MA, Dolmage TE. Influence of noninvasive positive pressure ventilation on inspiratory muscles. Chest 1991;99:408-415.

12. Bach JR, Campagnolo DI, Hoeman S. Life satisfaction of individuals with Duchenne muscular dystrophy using long-term mechanical ventilatory support. Am J Phys Med Rehabil 1991;70:129-135.

13. Paulus J, Willig TN. Nasal ventilation in neuromuscular disorders: respiratory management and patients' experience. Eur Respir Rev 1993;3:245-250.

14. Roussos C. Function and fatigue of respiratory muscles. Chest 1985;88:124S-132S.

15. Hill NS, Eveloff SE, Carlisle CC, et al. Efficacy of nocturnal nasal ventilation in patients with restrictive thoracic disease. Am Rev Respir Dis 1992;101:516-521.

16. Mohr CH, Hill NS. Long-term follow-up of nocturnal ventilatory assistance in patients with respiratory failure due to Duchenne-type muscular dystrophy. Chest 1990;97:91-96.

17. Ellis ER, Grunstein RR, Shu Chan S, et al. Noninvasive ventilatory support during sleep improves respiratory failure in kyphoscoliosis. Chest 1988;94:811-815.

18. Bach JR, Alba AS, Saporito LR. Intermittent positive pressure ventilation via the mouth as an alternative to tracheostomy for 257 ventilator users. Chest 1993;103:174-182.

19. Braun NMT, Faulkner J, Hughes R, et al. When should respiratory muscles be exercised? (Clinical Conference) Chest 1983;84:76-84.

20. Leger P, Jennequin J, Gerard M, et al. Home positive pressure ventilation via nasal mask for patients with neuromuscular weakness or restrictive lung or chest wall deformities. Respir Care 1989;34:73-77.

21. Braun NM, Marino WD. Effect of daily intermittent rest of respiratory muscles in patients with severe chronic airflow limitation (CAL). Chest 1984;85:59S-60S.

22. Heckmatt JZ, Loh L, Dubowitz V. Night-time nasal ventilation in neuromuscular disease. Lancet 1990;335:579-582.

23. Juan G, Calverley P, Talamo C, et al. Effect of carbon dioxide on diaphragmatic function in human beings. N Engl J Med 1984;310:874-879.

24. Freyschuss V, Nilsonne U, Lundgren KD. Idiopathic scoliosis in old age. I. Respiratory function. Acta Med Scand 1968;184:365-372.

25. De Troyer A, Pride NB. The respiratory system in neuromuscular disorders. In Macklin R, Roussos C (eds). The Thorax. New York, Marcel Dekker, 1985, pp 1089-1121.

26. Pinto AC, Evangelisya T, Carvalho M, et al. Respiratory assistance with a noninvasive ventilator (BiPAP) in NMD/ALS patients: survival rates in a controlled trial. J Neurol Sci 1995;129(suppl):19-26.

27. Ström K, Pehrsson K, Boe J, Nachemson A. Survival of patients with severe thoracic spine deformities receiving domiciliary oxygen therapy. Chest 1992;102:164-168.

28. Robert D, Gerard M, Leger P, et al. La ventilation mécanique à domicile définitive par trachéotomie de l'insuffisant respiratoire chronique. Rev Fr Mal Resp 1983;11:923-936.

29. Robert D, Leger P, Gerard M, et al. Utilisation de l'oxygén therapie de longue durée en dehors des bronchopneumopathies chroniques obstructives. Agressologie 1988;29:525-528.

30. Vianello A, Bevilacqua M, Salvador V, et al. Long-term nasal intermittent positive pressure ventilation in advanced Duchenne's muscular dystrophy. Chest 1994;105: 445-448.

31. Leger P, Petitjean T, Langevin B, Robert D. Long term effects of nocturnal nasal positive pressure ventilation at home. In Robert D, Make BJ, Leger P(cds). Home Mechanical Ventilation. Paris, Arnette Blackwell, 1995, p 205.

32. Gay PC, Patel AM, Viggiano RW, et al. Nocturnal nasal ventilation for treatment of patients with hypercapnic respiratory failure. Mayo Clinic Proc 1991;66:695-703.

33. Aboussouan LS, Khan SU, Meeker DP, et al. Effect of noninvasive positive pressure ventilation on survival in amyotrophic lateral sclerosis. Ann Intern Med 1997;127:450-453.

34. Simonds AK. Nasal intermittent positive pressure ventilation in neuromuscular and chest wall disease. Monaldi Arc Chest Dis 1993;48(2):156-168.

35. Jimenez JFM, de Cos Escuin JS, Vicente CD, et al. Nasal intermittent positive pressure ventilation: analysis of its withdrawal. Chest 1995;107:382-388.

36. Annane D, Quera-Salva MA, Lofaso F, et al. Mechanisms underlying effects of nocturnal ventilation on daytime blood gases in neuromuscular diseases. Eur Respir J 1999;13:157-162.

37. Schonhofer B, Geibel M, Sonneborn M, et al. Daytime mechanical ventilation in chronic respiratory insufficiency. Eur Respir J 1997;10:2840-2846.

38. Ellis ER, McCauley VB, Mellis C, Sullivan CE. Treatment of alveolar hypoventilation in a six-year-old girl with intermittent positive pressure ventilation through a nose mask. Am Rev Respir Dis 1987;136:188-191.

39. DiMarco AF, Connors AF, Altose MD. Management of chronic alveolar hypoventilation with nasal positive pressure breathing. Chest 1987;92:952-954.

40. Bach JR, Brougher P, Hess DR, et al. Consensus statement: noninvasive positive pressure ventilation. Respir Care 1997;42:365-369.

41. Piper AJ, and Sullivan CE. Effects of short-term NIPPV in the treatment of patients with severe obstructive sleep apnea and hypercapnia. Chest 1994;105:434-444.

42. Sanders MH, Kern NB. Obstructive sleep apnea treated by independently adjusted inspiratory and expiratory positive airway pressure via nasal mask. Chest 1990;98:317-324.

43. Reeves-Hoche MK, Hudgel DW, Meck R, et al. Continuous versus bilevel positive airway pressure for obstructive sleep apnea. Am J Respir Crit Care Med 1995;151:443-449.

44. Pankow W, Hijjeh N, Schuttler F, et al. Influence of noninvasive positive pressure ventilation on inspiratory muscle activity in obese subjects. Eur Respir J 1997;10:2847-2852.
45. Muir JF, Bota S, Cuvelier A, et al. Acute respiratory failure and obesity: incidence of management with noninvasive mechanical ventilation. Am J Respir Crit Care Med 1998;157:A309.
46. Consensus Conference. Clinical indications for noninvasive positive pressure ventilation in chronic respiratory failure due to restrictive lung disease, COPD, and nocturnal hypoventilation: a Consensus Conference Report. Chest 1999;116:521-534.
47. Sanders MH, Kern NB, Costantino JP, et al. Accuracy of end-tidal and transcutaneous PCO_2 monitoring during sleep. Chest 1994;106:472-483.
48. Rideau Y, Gatin G, Bach J, Gines G. Prolongation of life in Duchenne's muscular dystrophy. Acta Neurol 1983;5:118-124.
49. Raphael JC, Chevret S, Chastang C, et al. French multicenter trial of prophylactic nasal ventilation in Duchenne muscular dystrophy. Lancet 1994;343:1600-1604.
50. Masa JF, Celli BR, Riesco JA, et al. Noninvasive positive pressure ventilation and not oxygen may prevent overt ventilatory failure in patients with chest wall diseases. Chest 1997;112:207-213.
51. Bach JR. Update and perspective on noninvasive respiratory muscle aids. Part 2: The expiratory aids. Chest 1994;105:1538-1544.
52. Bach JR, Ishikawa Y, Kim H. Prevention of pulmonary morbidity for patients with Duchenne muscular dystrophy. Chest 1997;112:1024-1028.
53. Branthwaite MA. Noninvasive and domiciliary ventilation: positive pressure techniques. Thorax 1991;46:208-212.

Chapter 8

Noninvasive Ventilation in Severe Stable Chronic Obstructive Pulmonary Disease

Mark W. Elliott, M.D., M.R.C.P., Nicholas S. Hill, M.D.

Introduction

Chronic obstructive pulmonary disease (COPD) is the most common cause of respiratory failure worldwide and is associated with considerable morbidity and mortality.[1,2] With continued high smoking rates throughout the world, this is likely to be the case for the foreseeable future. Pharmacological therapy of COPD aims to alleviate symptoms mainly by reversing airway obstruction, but in many patients, the obstruction is largely irreversible. In time, patients develop respiratory failure, pulmonary hypertension, and cor pulmonale. Once peripheral edema supervenes, the prognosis is very poor with a 5-year mortality rate between 70% and 100%.[3] Therefore, various alternative therapeutic strategies have been developed to treat the consequences of chronic airway obstruction in an attempt to reduce symptoms, improve functional status, and prolong survival. These approaches include long-term oxygen therapy (LTOT), respiratory stimulant drugs, mechanically assisted ventilation, and surgical approaches including lung volume reduction surgery and lung transplantation.

After a number of preliminary, uncontrolled studies of LTOT showed benefit, two large randomized controlled trials of domiciliary oxygen therapy were performed in the United States (Nocturnal Oxygen Therapy Trial [NOTT]) and the United Kingdom (Medical Research Council [MRC]).[4,5] Although their protocols differed, both showed significant reductions in mortality with LTOT. Based on these findings, domiciliary oxygen therapy is now the only therapy that has been

From *Noninvasive Positive Pressure Ventilation: Principles and Applications,* edited by Nicholas S. Hill. © 2001, Futura Publishing Company, Inc., Armonk, NY.

shown to improve survival of patients with chronic hypoxemia due to COPD in a randomized controlled trial and, as such, it is the gold standard for their treatment.

Nonetheless, there are a number of reasons for considering additional therapies. In the MRC trial, there was no survival advantage from oxygen until after 500 days of treatment had elapsed. During this period, before a demonstrable beneficial effect on survival, the best predictor of death (and therefore a lack of benefit from oxygen) was a combination of polycythemia and hypercapnia. Further, the NOTT study showed that changes in hematocrit were unrelated to survival. These observations suggest that hypercapnia may be responsible for the poorer prognosis and lack of response to oxygen therapy. Further evidence for this hypothesis comes from the study of Cooper et al.,[6] who showed that, although the benefit from oxygen was apparent immediately, 29 of their 57 hypercapnic COPD patients died during the course of the study compared with only 3 of 15 normocapnic patients. Although hypercapnia may merely be a marker for more severe disease in these patients, the findings raise the possibility that applying a therapy that lowers CO_2 in these patients could improve survival.

Another reason to pursue alternative therapies is that although compliance with LTOT was very good in the controlled trials, this is not always the case in routine clinical practice. The main reasons for noncompliance are the lifestyle restrictions imposed by the need for 16 hours of oxygen therapy per day, and unfounded fears that oxygen is "addictive." Symptomatic patients who benefit subjectively from O_2 therapy are more likely to comply with therapy, but asymptomatic patients tend to use oxygen for too little time to gain a survival benefit.[7,8] These limitations (Table 1) raise the possibility that a therapy that

---

Table 1
Clinical Aspects of Long-Term Oxygen Therapy

- Proven to improve survival in hypoxic COPD
    Medical Research Council and Nocturnal Oxygen Therapy Trials
    Slows increase in pulmonary vascular resistance
    Enhanced cerebral perfusion
- Compliance problems in routine practice
- Failure to reduce or may even contribute to greater hypercapnia
- Inconvenient and cosmetically unappealing
- Lack of subjective improvement in some patients
    May worsen symptoms of fatigue, somnolence, headache
    Possible adverse effect on survival if hypercapnia is enhanced

does not interfere with daily activity and reduces CO_2 tension may be better tolerated and enhance the survival benefit in COPD when compared with LTOT. With the observation that home noninvasive ventilation is effective in the management of patients with restrictive thoracic disorders, interest has intensified in its role in the much more numerous group of patients with COPD.

Pathophysiology of Ventilatory Failure in Severe Stable COPD

The effectiveness of assisted ventilation in restrictive chest wall disease is not surprising given that there is a primary abnormality of the respiratory muscle pump, and the patient's lungs are usually normal. Assisted ventilation directly replaces the function of the patient's ailing respiratory pump. The situation is very different in COPD wherein the primary abnormality lies in the patient's lungs, and the ventilatory pump is affected secondarily. Assisted ventilation does very little to alleviate the primary obstructive defect. However, a logical case can also be made for the extension of ventilatory assistance to severe stable COPD patients.

To understand why assisted ventilation improves gas exchange in patients with chronic respiratory failure, even during unassisted breathing, a basic understanding of the pathophysiology of ventilatory failure is required (Table 2). For breathing to be effective, the respiratory muscle pump must be able to sustain a sufficient level of ventilation against a given load. Neural drive from the respiratory center in the brain stem must also be intact. In other words, there must be a balance between load and capacity, with the system receiving adequate neural input. This is easily understood by considering the analogy of an individual attempting to carry a suitcase across a room. He may fail for a number of reasons:

- The suitcase may be so heavy that no one could carry it; i.e., the load is excessive.

- The individual may be too weak; i.e., the capacity is reduced.

- He may lack the necessary motivation and simply be too lazy; i.e., drive is lacking.

In the patient with COPD, all three of these components may be abnormal. Changes in load, capacity, and drive are neither "all

Table 2
Pathophysiology of Ventilatory Failure
and of Symptoms in Patients with Chronic COPD

Increased load
- Airway obstruction
- Inspiratory threshold load because of PEEPi
- Pulmonary hypertension

Reduced capacity
- Mechanical disadvantage due to hyperinflation
- Effects of hypoxia, hypercapnia, and acidosis upon muscle function

Reduced central drive
- Reduced chemosensitivity because of bicarbonate retention during sleep

Impaired sleep
- Quality impaired, possible contribution of hypoxia and hypercapnia
- Nocturnal desaturation, possibly important in genesis of pulmonary hypertension

PEEPi, intrinsic positive end-expiratory pressure.

or nothing" phenomenons nor are they static. Airway obstruction has a direct effect on load by increasing the impedance to inflation. It also leads to hyperinflation and may cause the development of intrinsic positive end-expiratory pressure (PEEPi) because alveolar emptying is incomplete at the end of expiration. (It is analogous to a balloon that is not allowed to deflate completely, leaving a positive pressure inside.) Inspiratory gas flow will only occur when the alveolar pressure falls below the pressure at the mouth and nose. Therefore, the presence of PEEPi requires that the first part of each inspiratory effort be wasted. Gas decompression must occur before any inspiratory air flow and this increases the work of breathing. This need to lower alveolar pressure before inspiration ensues is referred to as an inspiratory threshold load.

Other contributors to the respiratory muscle dysfunction of severe COPD include hyperinflation, which reduces capacity by forcing the intercostal muscles and diaphragm to shorten and thereby work at a mechanical disadvantage. The hyperinflation adds to the oxygen cost of breathing by necessitating the use of accessory muscles. Abnormalities of the pulmonary vasculature may also put a secondary load on the respiratory muscles by adding to dead space and increasing the minute ventilation needed to maintain gas exchange.

Gas exchange abnormalities also occur during sleep in many patients with severe COPD.[9,10] Ventilation is normally reduced during sleep because of blunting of the drive to breathe. A rise in $PaCO_2$ of up to 5–7 mm Hg is normal, but an excessive rise causes a transient acidosis that triggers a compensatory renal retention of bicarbonate. Repeated CO_2 increases can cause enough bicarbonate retention to reduce chemosensitivity to CO_2. A vicious cycle may ensue in which CO_2 retention leads to more bicarbonate retention, which begets more CO_2 retention.

Polysomnographic studies have also revealed frequent oxygen desaturations in patients with severe COPD, particularly during rapid eye movement (REM) sleep,[9,10] mainly related to alveolar hypoventilation. The rapid shallow breathing pattern that normally occurs during REM sleep exacerbates the increased dead space ratio of COPD patients and leads to an even greater decrease in alveolar ventilation than otherwise would be the case. In addition, hyperinflated patients depend more on intercostal and accessory muscle activity than do normal subjects. With the normal inhibition of intercostal and accessory muscle activity that occurs during REM sleep, the diaphragm alone is unable to maintain ventilation in hyperinflated patients.

The effect of these sleep-related derangements upon survival and daytime function is not well known. Nocturnal hypoxemia has been postulated to be important in the genesis of sustained pulmonary hypertension in COPD.[11] REM-related falls in oxygen saturation are associated with rises in pulmonary artery pressure of up to 20 mm Hg.[12] However, the effect of transient increases in pulmonary artery pressure during sleep is not clear. Higher mean pulmonary artery pressures and red cell masses were found in 36 patients with COPD and mild to moderate oxygen desaturations (desaturation to at least 85% and at least 5 min spent with an SaO_2 <90%) than in 30 patients who did not desaturate. However, the daytime oxygen saturations were also significantly different between these groups.[13] In humans, acidosis is also a pulmonary vasoconstrictor, and transient drops in pH related to rises in CO_2 during sleep may exacerbate the vasoconstrictor response to hypoxia.[14] Therefore, pulmonary hemodynamics could benefit more if not only hypoxia, but also hypercapnia was treated in patients with severe COPD.

Impaired sleep quality related to shortened total sleep time and frequent arousals is well recognized in COPD compared with age-matched controls.[15] Experience from patients with obstructive sleep apnea suggests that disrupted sleep is associated with impaired neuropsychiatric functioning and reduced quality of life. White et al.[16] showed that sleep-deprived normal subjects had blunted ventilatory responses to both hypoxia and hypercapnia and, therefore, impaired sleep quality may further reduce chemosensitivity in COPD patients. Investigators have provided conflicting results on the effect of LTOT on sleep quality in COPD patients, some showing an improvement,[17] and others, no benefit.[18] Although these studies did not monitor CO_2 tension, others have shown that a rise in $PaCO_2$ of 6–15 mm Hg is a reliable and powerful arousal stimulus,[19] more powerful even than severe hypoxemia (SaO_2 <70%).[20] This provides an additional rationale for assisting ventilation and attempting to control CO_2 retention in COPD patients: fewer arousals and improved sleep quality.

The pathophysiologic defects described above provide a strong rationale for the use of noninvasive ventilation in severe COPD, even though it has no direct effect on the primary defect of airway obstruction. It can lower the work of breathing by providing inspiratory assistance and counterbalancing auto-PEEP, improve nocturnal ventilation and enhance respiratory drive, thereby ameliorating daytime gas exchange defects, reduce the stimuli for pulmonary vasoconstriction and reverse cor pulmonale, and eliminate the stimuli for arousals during sleep, thereby improving sleep quality. Further, the experience in patients with chest wall deformity and neuromuscular disorders in whom correction of nocturnal breathing abnormalities results in improved daytime function, suggests that similar benefit might be achieved in COPD. In the following section, the evidence supporting the use of noninvasive positive pressure ventilation (NPPV) for severe stable COPD will be reviewed to determine whether the potential benefits have been demonstrated.

Evidence for the Efficacy of NPPV in Severe Stable COPD

Earlier experience with negative pressure devices in severe stable COPD was disappointing, with most patients tolerating the devices poorly, unable to use the equipment at home for as long as instructed or during sleep.[21] Subsequently, successful nasal positive pressure ventilation in severe stable COPD was reported in uncontrolled studies showing improved daytime blood gas tensions and sleep quality.[22,23] However, few controlled studies have been done and most of these have had small numbers of patients followed for relatively short periods of time. Strumpf et al.[24] performed a randomized crossover trial in 19 patients with COPD and found that 7 were unable to tolerate the nasal mask and an additional 5 withdrew because of intercurrent illness. Among the 7 patients who completed the trial, only tests of neuropsychiatric function improved significantly. No improvements in gas exchange, functional status, symptoms, gas exchange, or sleep quality occurred. Patients were initiated as outpatients with regular visits from a respiratory therapist. Adequacy of ventilation was confirmed during wakefulness by measurement of end-tidal CO_2 tensions, although this measure may be unreliable in patients with severe COPD. In addition, the patients were not particularly hypercapnic (mean $PaCO_2$ 46 mm Hg).

Meecham Jones et al.[25] also performed a crossover study of the use of nasal pressure support ventilation plus oxygen with oxygen alone and showed improved daytime arterial blood gas tensions, better quality sleep, and improved quality of life during the pressure support limb of the study. The improvement in daytime $PaCO_2$ correlated with a reduction in overnight transcutaneous CO_2.

Lin[26] studied 12 patients in a prospective randomized crossover study of no oxygen or NPPV, oxygen alone, NPPV alone, and oxygen plus NPPV, each for 2 weeks. There were no differences in tidal volume, minute volume, spirometry, diurnal arterial blood gas tensions, mouth pressures, or ventilatory drive. Sleep efficiency was worse during NPPV than with oxygen alone. However, the maximum tolerated inspiratory pressure averaged 12 cm H_2O and ranged from only 8 cm H_2O to a maximum of 15 cm H_2O. No data were given about the effect of NPPV on blood gas tensions during ventilation, and there was no statistically significant improvement in sleep hypoventilation with NPPV. Since the primary aim of noninvasive ventilation delivered during sleep is to control nocturnal hypoventilation, concerns must be raised about whether these inspiratory pressures were adequate to achieve the aim. Further, the 2-week trial period was probably inadequate to permit adaptation, explaining why patients slept less well during NPPV.

In an additional negative study, Gay et al.[27] screened 82 hypercapnic COPD patients for entry into a trial of NPPV versus sham ventilation, but only 13 were available for randomization after the others declined, were excluded because of comorbidity, or corrected their hypercapnia during a run-in period. Average initial $PaCO_2$ was 51 mm Hg. Of the 7 patients who received NPPV, only 4 completed the trial, and only 1 had a substantial reduction in daytime $PaCO_2$. All 6 patients in the sham group completed the trial and appeared to tolerate the device better. No significant differences were detected between the groups, but average inspiratory pressure in the NPPV group was 10 cm H_2O, so concerns about adequacy of ventilatory assistance must be raised with this study, as well. Table 3 lists possible reasons for the failure of the above studies to observe benefit with NPPV for severe stable COPD.

Two large retrospective analyses have examined the impact of NPPV on survival outcomes of patients with a variety of forms of chronic respiratory failure treated for periods ranging up to 5 years.[28,29] The major outcome variable in these studies was continuation rates of NPPV rather than survival per se, although the authors surmised that these closely paralleled one another. COPD patients in these trials were less apt to continue NPPV than patients with neuromuscular disorders or chest wall deformities, but the average duration of NPPV continuation for COPD patients was still 2–3 years. The continuation curve for NPPV was similar to the survival curve obtained for COPD patients treated with tracheostomy positive pressure ventilation as reported in an earlier long-term trial.[30] In addition, continuation of NPPV among COPD patients was comparable to survival curves for patients treated with continuous long-term oxygen therapy as reported in the NOTT.[5] In a more recent uncontrolled trial of 26 COPD patients who had increased hypercapnia with O_2 supplementation alone, nocturnal NPPV reduced daytime and nocturnal CO_2 tensions and improved survival over that seen in historical controls.[31]

These latter studies suggest that survival among COPD patients treated with long-term NPPV is at least as good as that of patients treated with tracheostomies or long-term oxygen therapy, but the retrospective and uncontrolled design of these trials greatly limits any conclusions that can be drawn. Two additional long-term trials used randomized controls but have only been reported in abstract form.[32,33] A European multicenter trial enrolled 123 patients with $PaCO_2$s averaging 56 mm Hg, randomized them to receive nocturnal nasal ventilation plus conventional therapy versus conventional therapy alone, and has followed them for an average of 4.3 years. A trend for improved survival

---

Table 3
Possible Explanations for Failure of Controlled Studies to Demonstrate Benefit of NPPV in Severe Stable COPD

- Patients not hypercapnic enough
- Insufficient inflation pressures to achieve adequate ventilation
- Effectiveness of control of nocturnal hypoventilation not confirmed
- Patients not sufficiently acclimatized to the technique
- Optimal outcome variables not selected
- NPPV ineffective in severe stable COPD

that was apparent on an earlier interim analysis among patients treated with NPPV has become weaker.[32] An Italian multicenter trial enrolled 115 COPD patients in whom $PaCO_2$ was > 50 mm Hg and showed no survival benefit after 2 years.[33]

Another outcome variable that may be favorably affected by long-term NPPV in COPD patients is the frequency and duration of hospitalizations and intensive care unit (ICU) admissions. After a hospitalization for an acute exacerbation, COPD patients are frequently rehospitalized, averaging almost 2 hospitalizations per patient for the next 6 months.[34] In their long-term follow-up study, Leger et al.[29] found that hospital days per year fell from 49 for the year before, to 17 for the year after, initiation of NPPV. More recently, Jones et al.,[35] in another retrospective analysis on patients who could not tolerate oxygen therapy alone, found that hospital days decreased from 16 days to 7 days for the years before and after initiation of NPPV. In addition, the preliminary reports from France and Italy both found significant reductions in hospital days/patient/years among NPPV-treated patients compared with controls.[32,33] Similarly, Vitacca et al.[36] found that ICU admissions for the year following NPPV treatment for COPD exacerbations averaged 0.12 compared with 0.3 for patients treated with invasive ventilation. These studies indicate that NPPV may be more effective in reducing the need for hospitalization than in improving survival. The mechanism to explain the reduction in the need for hospitalization has not been defined, but it may be related to stabilization of gas exchange abnormalities, or to the ability of patients to treat more COPD exacerbations in the home.

The above studies provide a "mixed picture" to support the use of NPPV in patients with severe stable COPD. Only one randomized, controlled trial has provided favorable results,[25] but each of the randomized trials that yielded unfavorable findings was flawed in one way or another, including small numbers, inadequate inspiratory pressures, or insufficient time to allow adaptation. There is little evidence to suggest that NPPV prolongs survival in severe COPD patients, but data from the uncontrolled trials provide stronger support for the idea that NPPV helps to avoid hospitalization. Based on currently available evidence, if NPPV benefits any subgroup of patients with severe COPD, it is likely to be those with severe daytime CO_2 retention and nocturnal hypoventilation such as those enrolled in the Meecham Jones study. This presumption notwithstanding, it is also clear that more evidence is needed in the form of randomized controlled studies before definitive conclusions regarding efficacy can be drawn.

One conclusion that can be drawn with confidence is that severe COPD patients acclimatize to NPPV with difficulty. In both of the large retrospective analyses from Europe, patients with COPD were much less likely to continue use of NPPV than patients with neuromuscular disease or chest wall deformities. Also, a recent study by Criner et al.[37] showed that only 50% of COPD patients were using NPPV after a year compared to 80% for patients with restrictive thoracic disorders despite in-patient initiation in a specialized respiratory care unit. These authors also observed a high need for adjustment in the mask and ventilator (in both, in approximately 35% of patients) during the acclimatization period, so close outpatient monitoring is advised after patients are discharged home.

How NPPV Works
to Benefit Patients with Severe COPD

An understanding of the pathophysiology of ventilatory failure and of the effects of sleep-disordered breathing is important both in selecting patients who are likely to benefit from noninvasive ventilation and also targeting the appropriate therapeutic outcomes. In the early studies of noninvasive ventilation in severe COPD, benefit was thought to derive from resting of chronically fatigued respiratory muscles (Table 4). A number of studies were performed during the mid-to-late 1980s to test this hypothesis. Most of these studies consisted of small numbers of patients who were often recovering from an acute exacerbation. Several studies found small increases in maximal inspiratory and expiratory pressures that have been cited as evidence of improved respiratory function. However, these studies were either uncontrolled[38,39] or very short term (3–7 days),[40-42] and did not consider the possibility that improved gas exchange,[43] and not necessarily muscle resting per se, might have been responsible for the improvements. However, others[44]

Table 4
Possible Mechanisms of Benefit for NPPV in Severe Stable COPD

- Rest of chronically fatigued respiratory muscles
- Resetting of central chemosensitivity to CO_2
    Increased excretion of bicarbonate
    Reversal of hypoventilation
- Improved sleep duration and quality

have reported improved daytime arterial blood gas tensions in the absence of changes in indices of respiratory muscle strength.

In an attempt to answer definitively whether respiratory muscle fatigue exists in severe stable COPD, Shapiro et al.[45] randomized 184 patients to active or sham negative pressure ventilation at home using a poncho wrap ventilator. There was no significant benefit in either group, but compliance with treatment was much less than anticipated. They also found no relationship between the primary end point, a 6-minute walk test, and the "dose" of respiratory muscle rest actually delivered, or between baseline characteristics such as hypercapnia or FEV_1 and the response to therapy. They concluded that respiratory muscle fatigue was not an important factor in the functional limitations of patients with severe COPD, and that little was to be gained by resting the respiratory muscles. However, their study did not exclude the possibility that some forms of noninvasive ventilation may be useful in severe COPD patients. Compliance with therapy was suboptimal in their study and the subgroup analyses lacked the necessary power to definitively exclude any significant relationships. Also, it is noteworthy that the mean $PaCO_2$ of the patients studied was only 44 mm Hg compared to mean $PaCO_2 > 50$ mm Hg for the negative pressure studies with favorable findings. Thus, the study did not exclude the possibility that hypercapnic patients may benefit from intermittent noninvasive ventilation.

The problems with patient compliance encountered in the longer-term studies using negative pressure ventilation compromise any firm conclusions about efficacy that can be drawn from these studies. On the other hand, it is fair to conclude that severe COPD patients do not comply well with negative pressure ventilation, probably even less well than with NPPV. If there was any potential beneficial effect of negative pressure ventilation on respiratory muscle function, it was outweighed by the disadvantages associated with the technique. These results have dampened enthusiasm for the use of negative pressure ventilation for severe stable COPD patients or for the use of any form of noninvasive ventilation for resting respiratory muscles.

In response to these findings, more recent studies have focused on the use of NPPV to control sleep-related hypoventilation as the primary therapeutic aim, with improvement in sleep quality as a secondary benefit. This approach posits that if the nocturnal rise in CO_2 can be prevented, bicarbonate retention will not occur. Indeed, if the CO_2 is lowered and a mild alkalosis is induced, bicarbonate will be excreted and chemosensitivity to CO_2 will be enhanced. In line with this idea, Berthon-Jones and Sullivan[46] showed a leftward shift of the ventilatory response curve to CO_2 in hypercapnic patients with severe obstructive sleep apnea after 90 days of treatment with continuous positive airway pressure (CPAP). In 8 patients with severe COPD ventilated noninvasively during sleep for 6 months, Elliott et al.[22] also showed a resetting of the ventilatory response to CO_2 in association with a reduction in serum bicarbonate and base excess.

As discussed earlier, COPD patients also have poor quality sleep associated with abnormal breathing patterns including hypopneas and hypoventilation, particularly during REM.[9,10] Nocturnal ventilatory assistance, by preventing episodes of greater hypoventilation has the potential of improving sleep quality. The Meecham Jones et al. study[25] suggests that this is the case, demonstrating a longer total sleep time during use of NPPV. Krachman et al.[47] and Elliott et al.[23] have also observed increases in sleep duration during nocturnal ventilatory assistance in COPD patients. However, NPPV also has the capability of contributing to arousals in association with air leaks,[48] and some investigators have observed decreases in total sleep time during NPPV use in patients with severe stable COPD.[26] If patients have substantial nocturnal hypoventilation, though, it is likely that on balance, NPPV improves sleep quality if the experience in patients with restrictive thoracic disorders has any relevance.[49]

Even if we accept that NPPV improves nocturnal hypoventilation and sleep quality in patients with severe stable COPD, this does not necessarily mean that these are the mechanisms by which NPPV works. Schonhofer et al.[50] have attempted to elucidate possible mechanisms of the sustained improvements in gas exchange seen after intermittent use of NPPV, at least on restrictive patients. In a carefully designed study, patients with neuromuscular disease or skeletal deformity were allocated to receive NPPV either during sleep or during daytime wakefulness for a 1-month period. In the awake group, patients were prevented from sleeping by having to respond to intermittent prompts from a signal generator. There were no differences between the two groups, each showing improved diurnal blood gas tensions, increased respiratory muscle strength, and increased central respiratory drive as evidenced by a slightly greater drop in inspiratory airway pressure at 0.1 sec. Overnight oxygen saturation and transcutaneous CO_2 tensions during spontaneous breathing were also improved similarly in both groups at the end of the study.

These results indicate that reversal of hypoventilation and excretion of bicarbonate, whether they occur during wakefulness or sleep, are important effects of NPPV. By analogy, if a bucket leaks during the night, the abnormality can be corrected by filling it up either during the day or at night. The fact that nocturnal and daytime assistance both achieve the same result does not mean that leak at night is not important. These results also indicate that although nocturnal ventilation is more convenient for the patient, individuals who are unable to tolerate NPPV during sleep may find that assisted ventilation by day is an acceptable alternative.

The potential mechanisms discussed above are by no means mutually exclusive, and in any given patient, one might be more important than another. Therefore, when administering NPPV to severe stable COPD patients, the ventilator should be set to reduce inspiratory muscle work, to achieve optimal synchrony so as not to contribute to arousals at night, and to augment ventilation so that bicarbonate excretion and resetting of respiratory sensitivity to CO_2 will occur. With these aims in mind, the following sections discuss patient selection and practical aspects of applying NPPV to COPD patients.

Selection of Patients with Severe Stable COPD to Receive NPPV

Because of the paucity of well-designed, randomized controlled studies with favorable findings, the selection of patients with severe stable COPD to receive NPPV has been a highly controversial issue.[51] Partly in response to aggressive marketing by home respiratory vendors and a rapid increase in billings for this application in the United States, the Health Care Financing Administration (HCFA), which determines reimbursement police for Medicare, has been reformulating reimbursement guidelines for the use of long-term NPPV in patients with severe COPD. In addition, a consensus group formed by the American College of Chest Physicians and the National Association of Medical Directors of Respiratory Care has recently provided recommendations for this application.[52] The latter group recommended that NPPV be considered for severe stable COPD patients who remain symptomatic despite optimization of other therapies including oxygen (Table 5).

Based on the previously discussed evidence, the consensus group recommended that patients with hypercapnia be considered for a trial of NPPV if $PaCO_2$ was > 54 mm Hg. If $PaCO_2$ was between 50 and 54 mm Hg, a trial of NPPV was recommended if sustained oxygen desaturation was detected (consistent with nocturnal hypoventilation) on an overnight oximetry despite oxygen supplementation. Acknowledging the difficulty in obtaining formal sleep polysomnography without an undue delay at many centers, the consensus group recommended polysomnography only for patients with a high suspicion for obstructive

Table 5
Consensus Conference Recommendations
for Use of NPPV in Severe Stable COPD*

1. Severe COPD documented according to American Thoracic Society guidelines and persisting symptoms despite optimal medical therapy including oxygen, and
2. Daytime $PaCO_2 \geq 55$ mm Hg in clinically stable patient, or
3. If $PaCO_2$ is 50–54 mm Hg and evidence of nocturnal hypoventilation, or
4. Repeated hospitalizations in setting of severe airway obstruction, and
5. Obstructive sleep apnea excluded.

*Adapted from reference 52.

sleep apnea, such as those with loud snoring who are overweight and have daytime hypersomnolence. They also recommended NPPV for patients with repeated hospitalizations for COPD exacerbations.

The guidelines formulated by HCFA parallel the recommendations of the consensus group, but at this writing, they require a $PaCO_2$ of at least 52 mm Hg and overnight oximetry showing a sustained desaturation while on the patient's usual oxygen therapy before NPPV will be reimbursed. In addition, HCFA requires an initial trial of NPPV without a backup rate for the first 2 months, with the physician asserting that the patient has benefited and is using the device for at least 4 hours per 24 hours after the first 2 months of use. The latter requirement was added because the reimbursement for NPPV without a backup rate is considerably less than that for NPPV with a backup rate. The HCFA guidelines require that obstructive sleep apnea be "considered and excluded" and do not recognize repeated hospitalizations as an indication. These guidelines apply only to Medicare recipients and are likely to be modified as new information regarding the use of NPPV for severe stable COPD becomes available. Reimbursement guidelines differ between insurers and countries, but the guidelines formulated by the consensus group should suffice in most settings.

Another consideration for selection of patients to receive NPPV is that successful initiation requires patience and persistence, both on the part of patients and clinicians. Efforts at initiation of NPPV require a considerable amount of time and patient cooperation; thus, only patients who are motivated should be selected. The patient who is intolerant of an oxygen mask or who is noncompliant with medications or other aspects of the therapy is unlikely to persist with NPPV. To optimize the chances for success, the clinician should select patients not only according to the consensus guidelines, but also with the latter considerations in mind (Table 6).

Practical Considerations for Applying NPPV in Patients with Severe Stable COPD

Techniques for initiation of NPPV are discussed in more detail in Chapter 2. The following will focus on aspects pertinent to COPD patients, taking into consideration the mechanical ventilatory defects discussed earlier.

Choice of Ventilator

A wide variety of ventilators are available for patients with COPD. Both pressure- and volume-targeted devices have been shown to be

---

Table 6

Selections to Optimize the Likelihood of
Success of NPPV in Patients with Severe Stable COPD

Patient Selection
- On maximum effective treament for COPD
- Intolerant of oxygen because of symptomatic hypercapnia
- Deteriorating despite LTOT–intractable edema, frequent hospitalization
- Motivated
- Able to protect airway; no excessive secretions

Ventilator selection
- Volume- or pressure-cycled
- Local expertise and availability
- Patient preference
- Economical

Interface/head gear selection
- Patient preference
- Best fit
- Preferably nasal because of enhanced tolerability
- Full face mask if incorrigible mouth breather or poor fit or excessive mouth leaks with nasal mask

Ventilator settings selection
- To achieve adequate control of nocturnal hypoventilation (confirmed by overnight monitoring)
- To minimize respiratory muscle activity (confirmed by observation)
- Inspiratory pressure initially 8–12 cm H_2O and increased gradually as tolerated to alleviate respiratory distress
- Expiratory pressure 4–5 cm H_2O initially, increased up to 7–8 cm H_2O if needed to enhance triggering
- Inspiratory flow rate at least 60 L/min

effective in improving arterial blood gas tensions.[53-55] In large measure, local familiarity, expertise, and availability, as well as patient comfort determine the choice (Table 6). With pressure-targeted ventilators, volume delivery depends on the impedance to air flow. If there is a leak in the circuit, flow will increase to compensate, but if there is airway obstruction or compliance is low, volume delivery will be reduced. With volume-targeted ventilators, a fixed tidal or minute volume will be delivered regardless of mechanical properties of the lung. If impedance to inflation is high, pressure is increased as needed up to some predetermined limit to assure delivery of the preset volume. However, if there is a leak, there will be no increase in inspiratory flow to compensate. With these considerations in mind, it is apparent that both modes of ventilation have features that may be advantageous in COPD patients; the capability of maintaining gas delivery despite changes in lung impedance with volume-targeted ventilators, and the capability of compensating for air leaks with pressure-targeted ventilators. Thus, either type of ventilator mode can be used.

Several studies have directly compared the two modes. Restrick et al.[53] found no difference in overnight oxygenation when the two ventilator modes were compared, but the effect on overnight CO_2 was not determined. Schonhofer et al.[55] compared 1 month each of pressure-targeted with volume-targeted ventilation in 30 consecutive patients, including 3 with COPD, requiring home mechanical ventilation. Most patients could be adequately ventilated using either mode, but 10 were deemed to be nonresponders to pressure-controlled ventilation because of immediate symptomatic deterioration (n=3) or a decline in symptom scores or PaO_2 (n=7) after 1 month. These patients were later successfully ventilated with volume-targeted ventilators. Nonresponders to pressure-targeted ventilation reported significantly more dyspnea, less mobility, and worse sleep quality than during use of volume-targeted ventilators, suggesting that, in these patients, overnight ventilation was not adequate with pressure-targeted machines. Conversely, Smith and Shneerson[56] observed an improvement in diurnal blood gas tensions in 10 patients who were switched from a volume-targeted to a pressure-targeted ventilator. In addition, some studies suggest that pressure-targeted devices are more comfortable for the patient.[57,58]

Pressure support has the capability of synchronizing well with patient breathing effort and avoids sudden increases in airway pressure that may occur with volume-targeted ventilation during coughing or swallowing. Also, the facility to add PEEP (or expiratory positive airway pressure [EPAP]) is an important consideration if triggering is to be optimized. Thus, pressure support is generally considered the mode of first choice, although patient-ventilator synchrony can pose problems.[59]

Choice of Interface

An ever increasing variety of masks are now commercially available and it is usually possible to find a suitable mask. Occasionally, a customized mask is required, but these may be expensive and require expertise for proper application. The major choice is between a nasal or oronasal "full" face mask. A nasal mask is usually more comfortable for chronic applications, but some patients with COPD are mouth breathers and may find it difficult to breathe exclusively through the nose (Table 6). On the other hand, full face masks are more apt to precipitate claustrophobic reactions, have a larger dead space that may impede CO_2 clearance, and may interfere with expectoration. Thus, either mask usually suffices, but if problems are encountered with one, a trial of the other may be warranted. In addition, patient characteristics like patency of the nares and quantity of secretions should be considered in making the initial choice.

Choice of Ventilator Settings

The more sophisticated ventilators offer a wide array of selections including inspiratory and expiratory duration, inspiratory and expiratory trigger sensitivities and the pattern of delivery of gas flow (rise time), whereas simpler devices allow only inspiratory and expiratory pressures to be set by the operator. Most ventilators offer a choice between timed modes, in which breaths are triggered by a timer independent of the patient's inspiratory efforts, a spontaneous mode in which ventilator breaths are triggered by the patient's inspiratory efforts, or an assist/control mode in which the two modes are combined. Although the need for a backup rate has not been established, the inclusion of a spontaneous mode is desirable to enhance patient-ventilator synchrony. This is because COPD patients may have quite irregular patterns of breathing during the transition from wakefulness to sleep and during REM sleep. In this context, it is noteworthy that Meecham Jones et al.[25] and Elliott et al.[23] used such ventilators, whereas Strumpf et al.[24] used the timed mode.

Once a mode is chosen, the next priority should be to match the ventilator's output with the patient's pattern of breathing. This is done by asking the patient about their preferences and by operator observation. Minor further adjustments can then be made in response to arterial blood gas tensions and the results of overnight monitoring. The inspiratory pressure is set to relieve dyspnea and to avoid excessive discomfort from the air pressure, usually in the 8–12 cm H_2O range to start. The selection of PEEP or EPAP level is particularly important in patients with COPD because of the patient-ventilator asynchrony caused by PEEPi. This may increase the work of breathing[60] and contribute to patient discomfort. Measurement of PEEPi is impractical in most clinical situations, but the level of extrinsic PEEP can be titrated against patient comfort and to reduce the degree of ventilator/patient asynchrony. As a rough rule of thumb, it should not be higher than 7–8 cm H_2O, although this recommendation is not based on any published data.

Monitoring

In addition to relief of symptoms, improvement in gas exchange is one of the major aims of assisted ventilation in patients with severe stable COPD, so effective ventilation must be confirmed by measurement of arterial blood gas tensions during wakefulness once the patient is comfortable and acclimatized to the ventilator. Settings can then be further adjusted depending on these results. It is also important to observe the degree of accessory muscle activation closely during these early stages to ensure that inspiratory effort is minimized. Upward adjustments in inspiratory positive airway pressure (IPAP) or EPAP may alleviate vigorous inspiratory efforts, enhancing patient comfort. Once satisfactory gas exchange has been achieved during wakefulness and the patient is sleeping while using the ventilator, adequacy of nocturnal ventilation should be confirmed by overnight monitoring. Monitoring of oxygen saturation may be helpful to assess gas exchange at night, but considerable hypoventilation may be obscured by oxygen supplementation. Arterial blood gas monitoring remains the gold standard for assessment of gas exchange, but may be impractical. Monitoring of transcutaneous CO_2 may be helpful as a way to detect trends in CO_2 retention, but end-tidal CO_2 is not a reliable measure in patients with severe airway disease.

Acclimatization to NPPV in Patients with COPD

Most COPD patients require time and support from the nursing and/or technical staff while they acclimatize to the ventilator. Time and patience at this stage are usually well rewarded because a hurried approach compromises patient confidence and a much greater investment of time and effort will be required later. During acclimation, most patients are apprehensive about the mask, headgear, and ventilator, and the sensation of air pressure is initially uncomfortable. The patient should be reassured that most individuals find this stage difficult. It is important during these early stages that the patient feel in control and not overtaken by a machine.

Good mask fit is critically important and patients should be allowed to experiment with different masks so that they are aware of the choices available. They should be shown how to put the mask on and how to take it off and disconnect the tubing. Attention must also be paid to the headgear that allows the mask to seal correctly and comfortably; poorly fitting headgear can lead to an ill-fitting mask. When ventilation is tried for the first time, the headgear should be removed and the mask held in place by the patient. Once the patient is comfortable with the sensation of positive air pressure, the head straps can be applied. If the patient is apprehensive, the initial use of a handheld mouthpiece may help to build confidence. The ventilator is set to match the patient's inspiratory and expiratory pattern by asking the patient if they have enough time to breathe in and out and whether or not the breaths are coming too quickly. It is not uncommon for patients to complain that the machine is going too fast, when in fact all breaths are triggered.

Because there is no need for ventilation to be improved immediately, the ventilator should initially be set at a low pressure or flow, even if this is unlikely to be sufficient for adequate ventilation. Starting with high pressures will be uncomfortable and it is much easier to gain the patient's confidence if they are comfortable. Ventilation can be increased subsequently as the patient adapts, and as dictated by blood gas results. Patients should also be coached to disconnect the ventilator tubing and remove the mask if problems arise, and they should be given a plan to deal with potential crises. Although it is seldom necessary, practice of emergency drills helps to instill the feeling that the patient, and not the machine, is still in control. Initially, the patient may use the ventilator only for brief periods, but with practice and encouragement this is soon increased to several hours. When the patient is reasonably happy with daytime use, ventilator use during sleep should be encouraged. During the early adaptation period, frequent home checks by a skilled home respiratory therapist are helpful, because COPD patients in particular require frequent adjustments in mask fittings or ventilator settings and, typically, have a more difficult time with acclimatization than neuromuscular patients.[37]

Conclusions

The use of NPPV for patients with severe stable COPD remains a controversial topic. Some studies favor its application, but a number of unfavorable studies have also been published. At the present time, the consensus opinion is that patients with substantial daytime CO_2 retention and greater hypoventilation at night are the ones most likely to benefit. Patients who respond favorably are likely to experience improved nocturnal and daytime ventilation, greater duration of sleep, improved symptoms, and, perhaps, less need for hospitalization. However, definitive studies establishing efficacy or the patient population that should receive NPPV have not been done. To optimize the chances of success, careful patient selection, intensive familiarization and acclimatization, and adequate monitoring of therapeutic effect are vital. At the present time, NPPV should be reserved for appropriate patients who have failed conventional therapy, but a trial in motivated patients seems warranted because they have few other therapeutic options and, given the complexities and associated discomfort of NPPV, they are unlikely to continue in the absence of any beneficial effect.

References

1. Burrows B, Earle RH. Course and prognosis of chronic obstructive lung disease. N Engl J Med 1969;280:397-404.
2. Boushy SF, Thompson HK, North LB, et al. Prognosis in chronic obstructive pulmonary disease. Am Rev Respir Dis 1973;108:1373-1383.
3. Sahn SA, Nett LM, Petty TL. Ten year follow-up of a comprehensive rehabilitation program for severe COPD. Chest 1980;77(suppl):311-314.
4. Medical Research Council Working Party Report. Long term domiciliary oxygen therapy in chronic hypoxic cor pulmonale complicating chronic bronchitis and emphysema. Lancet 1981;1:681-685.
5. Nocturnal Oxygen Therapy Trial Group. Continuous or nocturnal oxygen therapy in hypoxaemic chronic obstructive lung disease, a clinical trial. Ann Intern Med 1980;93:391-398.
6. Cooper CB, Waterhouse J, Howard P. Twelve year clinical study of patients with hypoxic cor pulmonale given long term domiciliary oxygen therapy. Thorax 1987;42:105-110.
7. Baudouin SV, Waterhouse JC, Tahtamouni T, et al. Long term domiciliary oxygen treatment for chronic respiratory failure reviewed. Thorax 1990;45:195-198.
8. Walshaw MJ, Lim R, Evans CC, Hind CRK. Factors influencing compliance of patients using oxygen concentrators for long-term home oxygen therapy. Respir Med 1990;84:331-333.

9. Douglas NJ, Calverley PMA, Leggett RJE, et al. Transient hypoxaemia during sleep in chronic bronchitis and emphysema. Lancet 1979;1:1-4.

10. Fletcher EC, Gray BA, Levin DC. Nonapneic mechanisms of arterial oxygen desaturation during rapid-eye-movement sleep. J Appl Physiol 1983;54:632-639.

11. Boysen PG, Block AJ, Wynne JW, et al. Nocturnal pulmonary hypertension in patients with chronic obstructive pulmonary disease. Chest 1979;76:536-542.

12. Coccagna G, Lugaresi E. Arterial blood gases and pulmonary and systemic arterial pressure during sleep in chronic obstructive pulmonary disease. Sleep 1978;1:117-124.

13. Fletcher EC, Luckett RA, Miller T, et al. Pulmonary vascular hemodynamics in chronic lung disease patients with and without oxyhemoglobin desaturation during sleep. Chest 1989;95:757-764.

14. Emery CJ, Sloan PJ, Mohammed FH, Barer GR. The action of hypercapnia during hypoxia on pulmonary vessels. Bull Eur Physiopathol Respir 1977;13:763-776.

15. Arand DL, McGinty DJ, Littner MR. Respiratory patterns associated with hemoglobin desaturation during sleep in chronic obstructive pulmonary disease. Chest 1981;80:183-190.

16. White DP, Douglas NJ, Pickett CK, et al. Sleep deprivation and control of ventilation. Am Rev Respir Dis 1983;128:984-986.

17. Calverley PMA, Brezinova V, Douglas NJ, et al. The effect of oxygenation on sleep quality in chronic bronchitis and emphysema. Am Rev Respir Dis 1982;126:206-210.

18. Fleetham JA, West P, Mezon B, et al. Sleep, arousals, and oxygen desaturation in COPD. Am Rev Respir Dis 1982;126:429-433.

19. Hedemark L, Kronenberg R. Ventilatory responses to hypoxia and CO_2 during natural and flurazepam induced sleep in normal adults (abstract). Am Rev Respir Dis 1981;123:190.

20. Berthon-Jones M, Sullivan CE. Ventilatory and arousal responses to hypoxia in sleeping humans. Am Rev Respir Dis 1982;125:632-639.

21. Zibrak JD, Hill NS, Federman ED, et al. Evaluation of intermittent long-term negative pressure ventilation in patients with severe chronic obstructive pulmonary disease. Am Rev Respir Dis 1988;138:1515-1518.

22. Elliott MW, Mulvey DA, Moxham J, et al. Domiciliary nocturnal nasal intermittent positive pressure ventilation in COPD: mechanisms underlying changes in arterial blood gas tensions. Eur Respir J 1991;4:1044-1052.

23. Elliott MW, Simonds AK, Carroll MP, et al. Domiciliary nocturnal nasal intermittent positive pressure ventilation in hypercapnic respiratory failure due to chronic obstructive lung disease: effects on sleep and quality of life. Thorax 1992;47:342-348.

24. Strumpf DA, Millman RP, Carlisle CC, et al. Nocturnal positive-pressure ventilation via nasal mask in patients with severe chronic obstructive pulmonary disease. Am Rev Respir Dis 1991;144:1234-1239.

25. Meecham Jones DJ, Paul EA, Jones PW, Wedzicha JA. Nasal pressure support ventilation plus oxygen compared with oxygen therapy alone in hypercapnic COPD. Am J Respir Crit Care Med 1995;152:538-544.

26. Lin CC. Comparison between nocturnal nasal positive pressure ventilation combined with oxygen therapy and oxygen monotherapy in patients with severe COPD. Am J Respir Crit Care Med 1996;154:353-358.

27. Gay P, Hubmayr RD, Stroetz RW. Efficacy of nocturnal nasal ventilation in stable, severe chronic obstructive pulmonary disease during a 3-month controlled trial. Mayo Clin Proc 1996;71:533-542.

28. Simonds AK, Elliott MW. Outcome of domiciliary nasal intermittent positive pressure ventilation in restrictive and obstructive disorders. Thorax 1995;50:604-609.

29. Leger P, Bedicam JM, Cornette A, et al. Nasal intermittent positive pressure ventilation: long-term follow-up in patients with severe chronic respiratory insufficiency. Chest 1994;105:100-105.

30. Robert D, Gerard M, Leger P, et al. La ventilation mechanique a domicile definitive par tracheostomie de l'insuffisant respiratoir chronique. Rev Fr Mal Resp 1983;11:923-936.

31. Sivasothy P, Smith IE, Shneerson JM. Mask intermittent positive pressure ventilation in chronic hypercapnic respiratory failure due to chronic obstructive pulmonary disease. Eur Respir J 1998;11:34-40.

32. Muir JF, De La Salmoniere P, Cuvelier A, et al. Survival of severe hypercapnic COP/D under long-term home mechanical ventilation with NIPPV + oxygen versus oxygen therapy alone: preliminary results of a European multicenter study. Am J Respir Crit Care Med 1999;A295.

33. Clini E, Sturani C. The Italian multicenteric study of noninvasive nocturnal pressure support ventilation (NPSV) in COPD patients. Am J Resp Crit Care Med 1999;259:A295.

34. Connors AF, Dawson NV, Thomas C, et al. Outcomes following acute exacerbation of severe chronic obstructive lung disease. Am J Respir Crit Care Med 1996;154:959-967.

35. Jones SE, Packham S, Hebden M, Smith AP. Domiciliary nocturnal intermittent positive pressure ventilation in patients with respiratory failure due to severe COPD: long term follow up and effect on survival. Thorax 1998;53:495-498.

36. Vitacca M, Clini E, Rubini F, et al. Noninvasive mechanical ventilation in severe chronic obstructive lung disease and acute respiratory falure: short and long-term prognosis. Intensive Care Med 1996;22:94-100.

37. Criner GJ, Brennan K, Travaline JM, Kreimer D. Efficacy and compliance with noninvasive positive pressure ventilation in patients with chronic respiratory failure. Chest 1999;116:667-675.

38. Braun NM, Marino WD. Effect of daily intermittent rest of respiratory muscles in patients with severe chronic airflow limitation (CAL). Chest 1984;85:59S-60S.

39. Gutierrez M, Berolza T, Contreras G, et al. Weekly cuirass ventilation improves blood gases and inspiratory muscle strength in patients with chronic air-flow limitation and hypercarbia. Am Rev Respir Dis 1988;138:617-623.

40. Cropp A, Dimarco AF. Effects of intermittent negative pressure ventilation on respiratory muscle function in patients with severe chronic obstructive pulmonary disease. Am Rev Respir Dis 1987;135:1056-1061.

41. Scano G, Gigliotti F, Duranti R, et al. Changes in ventilatory muscle function with negative pressure ventilation in patients with severe COPD. Chest 1990;97:322-327.
42. Ambrosino N, Nava S, Bertone P, et al. Physiologic evaluation of pressure support ventilation by nasal mask in patients with stable COPD. Chest 1992;101:385-391.
43. Juan G, Calverley P, Talamo C, et al. Effect of carbon dioxide on diaphragmatic function in human beings. N Engl J Med 1984;310:874-879.
44. Barbe F, Quera-Salva MA, de Lattre J, et al. Long-term effects of nasal intermittent positive pressure ventilation on pulmonary function and sleep architecture in patients with neuromuscular diseases. Chest 1996;110:1179-1183.
45. Shapiro SH, Ernst P, Gray-Donald K, et al. Effect of negative pressure ventilation in severe chronic obstructive pulmonary disease. Lancet 1992;340:1425-1429.
46. Berthon-Jones M, Sullivan CE. Time course of change in ventilatory response to CO_2 with long-term CPAP therapy for obstructive sleep apnea. Am Rev Respir Dis 1987;135:144-147.
47. Krachman SL, Quaranta AJ, Berger TJ, Criner GJ. Effects of noninvasive positive pressure ventilation on gas exchange and sleep in COPD patients. Chest 1997;112:623-628.
48. Meyer TJ, Pressman MR, Benditt J, et al. Air leaking through the mouth during nocturnal nasal ventilation: effect on sleep quality. Sleep 1997;20:561-569.
49. Jimenez JFM, de Cos Escuin JS, Vicente CD, et al. Nasal intermittent positive pressure ventilation: analysis of its withdrawal. Chest 1995;107:382-388.
50. Schonhofer B, Geibel M, Sonnerborn M, et al. Daytime mechanical ventilation in chronic respiratory insufficiency. Eur Respir J 1997;10:2840-2846.
51. Rossi A, Hill NS. Noninvasive ventilation has been shown to be effective/ineffective in stable COPD: pro-con debate. Am J Respir Crit Care Med 2000;161:688-691.
52. Consensus Conference. Clinical indications for noninvasive positive pressure ventilation in chronic respiratory failure due to restrictive lung disease, COPD, and nocturnal hypoventilation: a Consensus Conference report. Chest 1999;116:521-534.
53. Restrick LJ, Fox NC, Braid G, et al. Comparison of nasal pressure support ventilation with nasal intermittent positive pressure ventilation in patients with nocturnal hypoventilation. Eur Respir J 1993;6:364-370.
54. Meecham Jones DJ, Wedzicha JA. Comparison of pressure and volume preset nasal ventilator systems in stable chronic respiratory failure. Eur Respir J 1993;6:1060-1064.
55. Schonhofer B, Sonnerborn M, Haidl P, et al. Comparison of two different modes for noninvasive mechanical ventilation in chronic respiratory failure: volume versus pressure controlled device. Eur Respir J 1997;10:184-191.
56. Smith IE, Shneerson JM. Secondary failure of nasal intermittent positive pressure ventilation using the Monnal D: effects of changing ventilator. Thorax 1997;52:89-91.

57. Vitacca M, Rubini F, Foglio K, et al. Noninvasive modalities of positive pressure ventilation improved the outcome of acute exacerbations in COLD patients. Intensive Care Med 1993;19:450-455.
58. Girault C, Richard J-C, Chevron V, et al. Comparative physiologic effects of noninvasive assist-control and pressure support ventilation in acute hypercapnic respiratory failure. Chest 1997;111:1639-1648.
59. Calderini E, Confalonieri M, Puccio PG, et al. Patient-ventilator asynchrony during noninvasive ventilation: the role of expiratory trigger. Intensive Care Med 1999;25:662-667.
60. Appendini L, Patessio A, Zanaboni S, et al. Physiologic effects of positive end-expiratory pressure and mask pressure suport during exacerbations of chronic obstructive pulmonary disease. Am J Respir Crit Care Med 1994;149:1069-1076.

Chapter 9

Application of Noninvasive Positive Pressure Ventilation in Children

W. Gerald Teague, M.D., David M. Lang, M.D.

Introduction

Noninvasive positive pressure ventilation (NPPV) can be an effective alternative to traditional therapies in pediatric-age patients with both acute and chronic respiratory system dysfunctions.[1] An important reason why NPPV should be considered in younger patients with acute respiratory symptoms is, in part, the high morbidity and mortality rates associated with endotracheal intubation and mechanical ventilation. Children with chronic respiratory failure are typically managed long term with a tracheostomy and assisted ventilation via volume-regulated ventilators. This therapeutic approach is fraught with a number of potentially serious complications, both medical and social. As a result, even though few published studies support the use of NPPV as a treatment for pediatric respiratory diseases, application of NPPV in younger patients is keeping pace with its growing use in adults.

Other factors contributing to the growing popularity of NPPV in the pediatric population are the relative ease and convenience of applying NPPV compared with the traditional invasive techniques. Also, the availability of soft nasal masks in a range of pediatric sizes and the introduction of portable pressure-targeted ventilators amenable to home use have encouraged greater use of NPPV. However, important differences between children and adults in the anatomy and mechanical function of the respiratory system as well as the spectrum of diseases causing respiratory failure bear on the application of NPPV in the pediatric-age patient. In the following, these differences will be considered, along with principles of pediatric patient selection and practical aspects of application.

From *Noninvasive Positive Pressure Ventilation: Principles and Applications,* edited by Nicholas S. Hill. © 2001, Futura Publishing Company, Inc., Armonk, NY.

Anatomic and Mechanical Features of the Developing Upper Airway

With few exceptions, NPPV is accomplished in children via a nasal mask interface. If this route of application is to be successful in augmenting alveolar ventilation, the resistance of the upper airway must be overcome. Important anatomic and mechanical features of the developing upper airway should be considered in the application of NPPV to pediatric patients since a relatively high inspiratory pressure setting may be necessary to overcome a high upper airway resistance (Table 1).

During infancy, resistance of the nasal airway is relatively high, and is a significant fraction of the total pulmonary resistance.[2] In young children, the nasopharyngeal airway is prone to obstruction for a number of reasons. The adenoids and tonsils develop naturally between 2 and 7 years of age and can enlarge in response to recurrent infections and allergies. Adenotonsillar hypertrophy is the most important cause of obstructive sleep apnea in the pediatric population. In addition, thick copious secretions can obstruct the nasopharyngeal airway in children with respiratory tract infections.

The size and shape of the nasopharyngeal airway are chiefly determined by the development of the midfacial bones.[3] Congenital craniofacial anomalies with maxillary hypoplasia such as those which occur with Down syndrome are often associated with obstructive sleep apnea or, in severe cases, obstructive hypoventilation syndrome. Young infants with choanal atresia or mandibular hypoplasia (Pierre Robin

---

Table 1

Factors Causing Obstruction of the Upper Airway and Limiting the Efficacy of NPPV via Nasal Mask in Pediatric Patients

---

- The nasal resistance is a relatively higher fraction of the total respiratory system resistance in pediatric patients than in adults.
- Acute nasopharyngeal obstruction with secretions often develops during upper respiratory infections.
- Adenoids and tonsils are relatively large and hypertrophic in response to respiratory infections.
- Congenital anomalies accompanied by maxillary hypoplasia can result in skeletal impingement on the nasopharyngeal airway.
- The larynx is in a relatively anterior location and there is a high incidence of conditions that promote laryngeal edema.
- The tendency to mouth breathe occurs as a compensatory response to nasopharyngeal obstruction.

anomaly) can also present with hypoventilation and severe respiratory distress.

Compared to the adult larynx, the immature larynx is positioned relatively anterior and contributes more to upper airway obstructive syndromes. Tonic activation of the laryngeal muscles during the first year of life produces an expiratory "braking mechanism," and thereby preserves lung volume. Infants and young children are more likely than adults to present with laryngeal airway obstruction in association with laryngomalacia, gastroesophageal reflux, and infectious laryngitis. Gastroesphageal reflux can cause laryngeal edema when acid reflux from the stomach reaches the larynx. NPPV may contribute to the tendency to have gastroesphageal reflux in children in situations where it contributes to gastric insufflation. However, the link, if any, between worsened gastroesophageal reflux and use of NPPV has not been established and gastroesophageal reflux is not a contraindication to NPPV in pediatric patients.

By necessity, children with obstruction of the nasopharyngeal airway mouth breathe in order to maintain adequate ventilation. However, this compensatory response may be counterproductive during nasal NPPV, when air leaking through the mouth can significantly limit the efficacy of NPPV.[4] Even though ventilators designed for NPPV are flow-triggered by the patient's respiratory effort, the onset of inspiration may be difficult to sense in the presence of large leaks. In addition, the duration of the inspiratory phase is dependent on the decrease in flow coincident with the attainment of the preset maximum inspiratory pressure. When the mouth leak is significant, patient inspiratory efforts may fail to trigger. If a backup rate is used, the timer will trigger inspiratory pressure, but inspiratory flow will be sustained in an attempt to maintain the inspiratory pressure, resulting in a prolonged inflation. The child may attempt to exhale during the inflation, giving rise to patient-ventilator asynchrony that is especially common in young children and infants who compensate for respiratory dysfunction by breathing rapidly.

Experience with NPPV in Pediatric Patients

The published clinical experience in pediatric-age patients treated with NPPV to date includes more than 100 infants and children (Table 2). All of the publications describing the use of NPPV in pediatric patients are case series that describe improvements in selected clinical variables over time. Presently, there are no published randomized con-

Table 2
Summary of Published Experience with NPPV via Nasal Mask in Pediatric Respiratory Diseases

Diagnosis	Study	Year	No. of Patients	Setting	Comments
Chronic failure with hypercarbia					
Central hypoventilation	Ellis et al.[6]	1987	1	Home	Improvement in ventilation.
Neuromuscular weakness	Nielson et al.[7]	1990	2	Home	CO_2 after 10 days use.
	Padman et al.[8]	1994	15	PICU	Effective in avoiding intubation.
Upper airway obstruction	Teague et al.[10]	1991	1	Sleep lab	Improved ventilation and SaO_2.
Cystic fibrosis	Piper et al.[11]	1992	4	Home	Reversed hypercarbia.
	Padman et al.[12]	1994	7	Home	In long-term use.
Bronchopulmonary dysplasia	Brown et al.[13]	1994	27	Home	Included 10 patients with BPD and tracheostomies.
Acute hypoxemic respiratory failure					
Pulmonary edema	Akingbola et al.[15]	1993	2	PICU	Reversed hypoxemia in two infants.
Hypoxemic respiratory failure	Akingbola et al.[16]	1994	9	PICU	Reduced FiO_2.
Pneumonia with hypoxemia	Fortenberry et al.[14]	1995	28	PICU	Acute improvement in oxygenation, low rate of intubation.
Acute asthma with hypoxemia	Teague et al.[18]	1997	26	PICU	Effective in most applications, but high rate of intubation.

PICU, pediatric intensive care unit.

trolled trials in support of NPPV as a standard treatment for any pediatric respiratory condition. However, the evidence in support of NPPV as a standard treatment is accumulating for a number of conditions involving adults, for example hypercarbic exacerbations of chronic obstructive pulmonary disease (COPD) (see Chapter 2).[5]

Among the first published pediatric applications of NPPV were reports of two 6-year-old children with chronic respiratory failure from congenital central hypoventilation syndrome (CCHS).[6,7] Standard therapies for these patients including mechanical ventilation via a tracheostomy, and diaphragmatic pacing are invasive and have a significant associated morbidity. These therapies were avoided by the successful application of nasal NPPV. However, NPPV has not been attempted in infants with CCHS. Therefore, NPPV should be reserved for older children with CCHS with supportive family members who choose this as an alternative to standard therapy. In those who already have tracheostomies, NPPV can be administered on a trial basis in the sleep laboratory or hospital with the tracheostomy capped under controlled conditions.

Long-term nocturnal use of NPPV is highly effective in pediatric patients with chronic respiratory failure from neuromuscular weakness or thoracic kyphoscoliosis.[8] In these patients, silent nocturnal hypoxemia with arousal during rapid eye movement (REM) sleep may occur months before daytime hypercapnia is evident. The sleep laboratory is an ideal location to both diagnose and treat children with respiratory complications associated with neuromuscular weakness.[4] Considering that treatment with supplemental oxygen may exacerbate CO_2 retention and is potentially dangerous, NPPV is a superior therapy in these patients in that it can also reverse hypoventilation while it reduces the load on the inspiratory muscles.

Children may develop nocturnal obstructive hypoventilation syndrome (OHS) as a complication of upper airway dysfunction, often in association with an underlying lung disease (Table 3). Such "overlap"

Table 3

Features of Obstructive Hypoventilation Syndrome

- Hypercarbia and hypoxemia associated with episodes of partial or complete upper airway occlusion during sleep.
- Thoracoabdominal asynchrony from prolonged activation of the respiratory muscles.
- Abnormalities most apparent during rapid eye movement sleep phase.
- Can complicate several types of respiratory dysfunction in pediatric patients.

syndromes are commonly seen in obese children and in patients with upper airway obstruction associated with cerebral palsy or craniofacial anomalies. The magnitude of the apnea-hypopnea index (AHI), commonly used to quantify the degree of nocturnal airway obstruction in adult patients, is not a sensitive indicator for the diagnosis of OHS in pediatric-age patients.[9] During prolonged episodes of partial airway occlusion, gas flow through the upper airway can be maintained through sustained activation of the respiratory muscles. NPPV is an ideal therapy in pediatric patients with OHS since the inspiratory pressure support feature on modern flow-triggered devices can "unload" the inspiratory muscles. We have found that NPPV does acutely improve respiratory gas exchange and reduce the number of airway occlusions in pediatric-age patients with OHS.[10] The efficacy of NPPV as a long-term therapy in OHS remains to be proven, although its potential as a bridge therapy to surgical correction of upper airway obstruction is promising.

NPPV has also been applied successfully in pediatric patients with cystic fibrosis complicated by hypercarbic respiratory failure as a bridge therapy to lung transplantation.[11,12] The benefit of NPPV in other pediatric diseases associated with severe airways obstruction, such as bronchopulmonary dysplasia (BPD), is less well defined. An important issue is whether portable flow-triggered pressure-targeted ventilators should be substituted for standard home ventilators in infants with BPD who have tracheostomies. Although the preliminary experience in one case series was promising,[13] we have found that gas leaks around the tracheostomy tube are a serious impediment to effective use of flow-triggered devices in such patients. The limited availability of nasal masks for small infants is another significant factor impeding application of NPPV in infants with BPD.

Experience with NPPV in pediatric-age patients with acute hypoxemic respiratory failure from pneumonia[14] or pulmonary edema[15,16] is also encouraging. In the two largest case series published to date,[14,16] NPPV consistently improved oxygenation, but its efficacy in reversing hypercarbia was less well established. Although the rate of endotracheal intubation in the largest series was low,[14] further experience is necessary before NPPV can be viewed as a reliable alternative to invasive ventilatory assistance in pediatric-age patients with acute hypoxemic respiratory failure complicated by hypoventilation.

NPPV via full face mask at low inspiratory pressures effectively improved respiratory gas exchange in critically ill adults with status asthmaticus,[17] but there is no published experience with the use of NPPV in children with status asthmaticus. We found in a preliminary report that NPPV via nasal mask in critically ill children with severe hypoxemia from asthma acutely decreased the respiratory rate, heart rate, and FiO_2 in a subset of patients who were managed without intubation.[18] However, we also found that a substantial proportion of children with status asthmaticus complicated by hypercarbia did not improve with NPPV and went on to require endotracheal intubation. Clinicians who attempt NPPV in children with acute hypoxemia from status asthmaticus should be aware of a relatively high rate of intolerance, mainly from agitation.

Indications for NPPV in Children

A number of respiratory conditions are amenable to a trial of NPPV in pediatric-age patients (Table 4). As a general principle, NPPV for chronic pediatric applications is likely to be most effective when applied intermittently to older children with stable disorders associated with alveolar hypoventilation. Such disorders include central hypoventilation syndromes, and chronic respiratory diseases associated with neuromuscular and chest wall impairment. It is prudent to bear in mind

Table 4
Respiratory Conditions Amenable
to a Trial of NPPV in Pediatric Patients

Restrictive Disorders	**Obstructive Disorders**
Duchenne's muscular dystrophy	Cystic fibrosis
Spinal muscular atrophy	Bronchopulmonary dysplasia
Mytonic dystrophy	Status asthmaticus
Thoracic kyphoscoliosis	Bronchiolitis obliterans
Overlap Syndromes	**Acute Hypoxemic Respiratory Failure**
Spina bifida	
Cerebral palsy	Pneumonia
	Acute chest syndrome in sickle cell
Obesity hypoventilation syndrome	Atelectasis
Obstructive hypoventilation syndromes	
	Postextubation Weaning
Impaired Central Respiratory Drive	
Congenital central alveolar hypoventilation	
Acquired central hypoventilation	
Infectious and metabolic encephalopathies	

that disorders associated with chronic hypoventilation may present in the very young. NPPV in this age group deserves consideration, but needs to be validated in further clinical trials. The application of NPPV for older children with obesity hypoventilation syndrome will likely become a standard therapy, preferred over nasal continuous positive airway pressure (CPAP) or long-term supplemental oxygen because of its capacity to increase tidal volume and improve CO_2 elimination.

Less certain is the role of NPPV in the management of respiratory dysfunction in pediatric patients primarily due to impaired ventilation/perfusion relationships. At this time, there is no evidence that NPPV has a role in such disorders in the very young other than its anecdotal use at home in infants with BPD.[13] For therapy of acute respiratory disorders, NPPV deserves consideration in pediatric patients with status asthmaticus and in disorders predominated by alveolar hypoxia, including acute pneumonia and acute pulmonary edema. However, the greatest value of NPPV in the acute setting may be to support patients with acute exacerbations of chronic disorders such as cystic fibrosis or bronchiolitis obliterans, when hypoventilation accompanies severe ventilation/perfusion derangement.

Practical Application in Children

Considerations for Initiation

The first step in initiating NPPV after selecting an appropriate pediatric patient is to decide on a location. The proper setting for a trial of NPPV depends on whether it is being used as a life support therapy (Type 1 application) versus a clinical benefit to enhance respiratory function (Type 2 application).[5] Life support applications of NPPV, i.e., those which, if withdrawn, would lead to imminent death, should not be attempted outside of the emergency room, recovery room, or intensive care unit. The appropriate setting should also be one that routinely handles unstable children with endotracheal tubes, mechanical ventilators, and intravenous sedation, and has practitioners skilled in the application of NPPV. Children treated with NPPV for life support indications must be closely monitored (Table 5). Contraindications to the use of NPPV as a life support therapy in children are similar to those that apply to adults and include cardiovascular instability, respiratory arrest, severe agitation, recent facial or gastrointestinal surgery, craniofacial trauma or burns, high aspiration risk, inability to protect the airway, and fixed anatomic obstruction of the upper airway.[5]

Table 5
Monitoring Requirements for NPPV
in Pediatric-Age Patients as a Life Support Therapy*

Patient
- Arterial blood gases
- End-tidal or transcutaneous CO_2**
- Continuous pulse oximetry
- Continuous respiratory and cardiac waveforms
- Systemic blood pressure
- Degree of respiratory distress
    Use of accessory muscles of respiration
    Location and severity of retractions
    Nasal flaring
- Breath sounds
- Physical evidence of gastric distension or subcutaneous emphysema
- Chest film

NPPV System and Mask Interface
- Airway pressures, including high and low pressure and disconnect alarms
- FiO_2
- Temperature of gas in the inspiratory circuit
- Serial charting of ventilator settings

* Removal from NPPV would result in imminent death.
** Utility has not been established.

In stable patients with chronic respiratory failure, NPPV can be safely initiated in settings such as a hospital general ward, sleep laboratory, or rehabilitation unit. Initiation at home may also be possible, depending on the comfort of the patient's parents and other caregivers with learning new techniques. In these settings, NPPV can be a transitional therapy that facilitates home care once the patient is familiar with the airway interface and the ventilator is adjusted optimally. Monitoring for children who undergo chronic applications of NPPV should include intermittent home visits by a respiratory therapist, symptoms, vital signs, and occasional daytime blood gases and nocturnal pulse oximetry. For patients in whom accidental removal from NPPV would result in significant hypoxemia, disconnect alarms and low pressure alarms should be included (Table 6).

Choice and Application of Interface

Soft nasal masks designed specifically for NPPV are available in a range of sizes and shapes for use in pediatric-age patients (Table 7).

Table 6
Monitoring NPPV Used
as a Clinical Benefit to Enhance Ventilatory Function

Patient
- Pulse oximetry*
- End-tidal CO_2*
- Cardiac and respiratory waveforms*
- Serial blood gas measurements of daytime $PaCO_2$ and forced vital capacity
- Anthropometric growth variables

NPPV System and Mask Interface
- Airway pressures and disconnect alarm*
- Ventilator timer for hours of use and patient tolerance

*Optional selections based on clinical status.

Table 7
Nasal Mask Dimensions for Pediatric NPPV*

Size	Width (cm)	Height (cm)
Small child	2.9	2.4
Petite	3.4	3.9
Small	3.6	4.6

*Available from Respironics, Inc., Murrysville, PA

The most important principle in mask selection is to be certain that it fits snugly around the perimeter of the nose. The masks are designed to fit from the bridge of the nose to just above the upper lip. Over-sized masks may appear to fit comfortably, but in fact require greater tension on the strap attachments to eliminate air leaks than do smaller masks. This can result in breakdown of the skin at the apex of the mask over the nasal bridge. The small child size (Respironics, Inc., Murrysville, PA) is relatively broad compared with other masks, conforming more to the unique facial structure of young children, and is recommended for patients as young as 1 year of age. This mask also includes a thin plastic "comfort flap," which fits between the mask and face to reduce air leakage and to improve comfort. Four sizes of forehead spacers that should be used to improve stability and reduce pressure on the nasal bridge are also included. Nasal pillows (or "seals") may be an effective alternative interface in older children who do not tolerate the standard nasal mask.

A full face mask suitably sized for pediatric NPPV is also commercially available (Respironics, Inc.). Face mask NPPV may be a suitable alternative to the nasal mask in children who mouth breathe or who have nasal obstruction or large mouth leaks. However, disadvantages of face mask NPPV in pediatric patients include the increased potential for claustrophobic reactions and a risk of aspiration of gastric material from vomiting. Experience with full face mask NPPV in pediatric patients is lacking at this time and deserves further study in specific clinical situations. It is likely not an appropriate interface for long-term use, especially in the very young.

Selection of a Ventilator

A number of so-called "bilevel" ventilators, compact, pressure-targeted, devices designed specifically to deliver NPPV, have become available for use in children. The advantages of these units over conventional volume-regulated ventilators include less weight for improved portability, better leak compensation, and the availability of inspiratory pressure support or pressure assist/control with or without positive end-expiratory pressure (PEEP). As a group, these ventilators are capable of providing variable and high initial peak flows.[19] Newer units feature an expanded inspiratory pressure range and an adjustable inspiratory pressure rise time. Because most of these units were designed for home applications, most lack an oxygen blender and lack an integrated airway pressure alarm.

Issues to consider in the selection of a pressure-targeted ventilator for pediatric use include the clinical indication, type of interface, potential for nasopharyngeal obstruction, the nature of the respiratory system dysfunction, and the possibility of mouth leaks. We do not recommend the use of portable pressure-targeted ventilators in patients with in-dwelling artificial airways unless methods to humidify the inspired gas and backup alarms are added. Considering that some older bilevel units had maximal pressure generating capabilities of 20 cm H_2O, for children who need higher inspiratory positive airway pressure (IPAP) levels, one of the newer pressure-targeted units or a volume-cycled unit should be selected (see Chapter 1). Tolerance and safety of NPPV by pediatric patients at pressures in this range have not been established.

Mouth leaks not infrequently limit the efficacy of NPPV in pediatric patients, especially those with severe respiratory distress. Options to reduce mouth leaks include chin straps, but these can agitate young children. The VPAP II S/T (ResMed Corporation, San Diego, CA), a recently introduced portable pressure-targeted ventilator, permits adjustment of the maximum IPAP duration. The potential advantage of this feature in diminishing the impact of mouth leaks is that it can prevent overly long inflations if the device fails to sense the onset of expiration. Thereby, the device enhances synchrony of the child's respiratory cycle with that of the ventilator. Further work with this unit is necessary in pediatric patients to see if it performs consistently better in this regard than other pressure-targeted devices.

Initial Settings

Recommended settings for the initiation of NPPV in pediatric-age patients should reflect the category of respiratory dysfunction and whether or not the child has a depressed ventilatory drive (Table 8). We typically initiate NPPV in pediatric patients at inspiratory pressures of 8–10 cm H_2O and an expiratory pressure of 4–6 cm H_2O. Children with central hypoventilation syndromes and depressed ventilatory drive must have a unit with a backup rate that will cycle in the absence of spontaneous respiratory effort. Relatively high IPAP levels may be necessary to improve gas exchange in children with obesity hypoventilation syndrome and other conditions that reduce respiratory system compliance or increase inspiratory airway resistance. In children with severe status asthmaticus and hypoxemia, we have found that NPPV at inspiratory pressures < 20 cm H_2O may improve oxygenation, but does not consistently reverse hypercarbia.[18]

Table 8
Recommended Initial Settings for NPPV in Pediatric Patients

Clinical Setting	Modes	IPAP (cm H_2O)	EPAP (cm H_2O)	Rate (# / min)
Disorders with hypoventilation				
Central hypoventilation	S/T or T	8–10	4–6	20
Neuromuscular disorders	S/T or T	8–12	4–6	20
Obesity hypoventilation syndrome	S/T or T	14–16	6–8	10–20
Disorders with ventilation/perfusion mismatch				
Pneumonia with atelectasis	S or S/T	10–14	6–8	10
Asthma with atelectasis	S/T or T	12–16	6–8	10

IPAP, inspiratory positive airway pressure; EPAP, expiratory positive airway pressure; S, spontaneous; S/T, spontaneous/timed; T, timed.

NPPV via a bilevel ventilator may not reduce a child's $PaCO_2$ when exhaled CO_2 does not clear the in-line exhalation valve or when the dead space of the nasal mask is large.[19] The problem with CO_2 rebreathing may be eliminated by raising the positive end-expiratory pressure (PEEP) level above 4 cm H_2O or substituting an isolated one-way exhalation valve in the ventilator circuit.[20] Higher expiratory positive airway pressure (EPAP) settings are also often necessary if patients have atelectasis, hypoventilation associated with ventilation/perfusion mismatch, or a component of obstructive sleep apnea.

With bilevel ventilation, the FiO_2 can be raised by connecting oxygen tubing to a port on the mask or a T-connection in the ventilator circuit. The problem with this method is that FiO_2 delivery is not precise. Alternatively, oxygen can be blended into the circuit by diverting the connection tubing between the pressure-targeted unit and nasal mask through a conventional heater/humidifier/oxygen source. This method has the advantages of conditioning the inspired gas and allowing some estimate of the FiO_2 via an oxygen sensor electrode in the circuit. However, since portable pressure-targeted ventilators deliver gas at very high flow rates, we have found that, in children with significant hypoxemia, a very high flow rate of supplemental oxygen is required to enrich the FiO_2. Patients with profound hypoxemia may be better served by oxygenation using a "critical care" ventilator with an oxygen blender.

Adaptation and Monitoring

The most important goals of NPPV with pressure-targeted ventilators in young patients are to alleviate respiratory distress, decrease the work of breathing, and maintain an acceptable comfort level. In children with acute respiratory distress, this is done primarily by raising the inspiratory pressure support level incrementally until the respiratory rate falls, retractions diminish, and there is less visible recruitment of the accessory muscles of breathing (Table 5). In most applications, the patient's $PaCO_2$ decreases coincident with a reduction in respiratory distress, but the change in $PaCO_2$ may be delayed, especially in very obese children[10] or in cases of severe status asthmaticus.[18] Typically, with most types of chronic hypercarbic respiratory failure in children, the $PaCO_2$ gradually decreases even at relatively low inspiratory pressures (i.e., 10–12 cm H_2O).

For patients with persisting hypoxemia despite high flow supplemental O_2, the expiratory pressure can be adjusted upward in 2 cm H_2O

increments until the SaO_2 is consistently above 90%. If an expiratory pressure exceeding 8 cm H_2O is required to maintain oygenation, switching to a ventilator with an oxygen blender that delivers accurate, high FiO_2 is recommended before increasing the expiratory pressure further. The sleep laboratory is useful for making these adjustments in the nonacute setting, because muscular hypotonia associated with REM sleep potentiates respiratory gas exchange abnormalities in children with chronic lung diseases, and the pressures and backup rate necessary to prevent these abnormalities can rapidly be determined.

Complications of NPPV in Children

Serious complications of NPPV in children are unusual and, in our experience, have been restricted to pneumothorax and pneumomediastinum in a single critically ill patient with status asthmaticus. Pediatric patients are prone to unique complications of NPPV based on a number of factors (Table 9). Because reflux and regurgitation are quite common in small children who may have a low gastroesphageal sphincter tone, gastric distension occurs frequently and may potentiate aspiration or gastroesophageal reflux in children who are being fed. In spite of this

Table 9
Potential Complications of NPPV Unique to Pediatric Patients

Complication	Factor Unique to Pediatric Patients
Aspiration of gastric contents	Immaturity of airway protective reflexes
Exacerbation of gastroesophageal reflux	Impaired gastroesophageal sphincter function in the very young
Increased upper airway obstruction	Reduced clearance of upper airway secretions
Conditions associated with anatomic laryngeal obstruction	Laryngomalacia
Asynchronous respiratory pattern	Tendency of children with upper airway obstruction to mouth breathe
Anxiety	Natural concern with new situations dependence on others for care
High incidence of developmental disorders	

risk, we have not seen serious aspiration pneumonia in children treated with NPPV, even in the presence of low-volume continuous feeds via a nasogastric tube.

Minor complications of NPPV occur commonly in children. The most frequent complaints are anxiety associated with mask placement, irritation of the skin at the mask margins, and nasal dryness. Nearly all of these can be reversed through selection of the appropriately sized nasal mask, skin care, and humidification of the circuitry. Working closely with the child, explaining each step of the procedure in advance, and gaining his/her trust can minimize anxiety. The likelihood of NPPV success is also increased when applied by staff who are experienced in working with NPPV in children with respiratory disorders.

Summary

Children with a variety of clinical disorders ranging from acute respiratory distress caused by pneumonia to chronic respiratory failure from progressive neuromuscular weakness can benefit from NPPV. In the acute setting, NPPV may be attempted as a therapy to prevent endotracheal intubation, but the child must be monitored in a unit that routinely handles pediatric patients with severe respiratory dysfunction. In children with chronic respiratory failure, nocturnal application of NPPV appears to be highly effective in improving respiratory gas exchange and is more adaptable to the home environment than mechanical ventilation via a tracheostomy. However, it has not been shown conclusively that NPPV prolongs survival as effectively as positive pressure ventilation via a tracheostomy in children with respiratory failure from advanced neuromuscular weakness. Also, the role of NPPV in BPD has not yet been established, although anecdotal evidence suggests that it can be used effectively.

The use of NPPV in the acute setting has not been established by controlled trials, either, although a number of case series suggest that it can be used to avert intubation in critically ill children with acute hypoxemic respiratory failure from status asthmaticus, acute respiratory distress syndrome, and acute chest syndrome. Further study will be necessary to determine which acutely ill pediatric patients are most likely to benefit from NPPV and how to select them. Technical limitations of NPPV that are present in adults but sometimes more challenging in children because of upper airway structural features and rapid breathing rates include persistent mouth leaks and patient-ventilator asynchrony. These impair the effectiveness of NPPV, but technical advances in the design of full face masks and second generation pressure-targeted ventilators are likely to reduce leak and improve patient comfort, facilitating the acceptability and efficacy of NPPV in pediatric patients, leading to expanded applications.

References

1. Teague WG. Pediatric application of noninvasive ventilation. Respir Care 1997;42:414-423.
2. Stocks J, Godrey S. Nasal resistance during infancy. Respir Physiol 1978;34:233-246.
3. Burstein F, Cohen S, Scott P, et al. Surgical therapy for severe refractory sleep apnea in infants and children: application of the airway zone concept. Plast Reconstr Surg 1995;96:34-41.
4. Piper A, Willson G. Nocturnal nasal ventilatory support in the management of daytime hypercapnic respiratory failure. Aust Physiother 1996;42:17-28.
5. Bach JR, Brougher P, Hess DR, et al. Consensus statement: noninvasive positive pressure ventilation. Respir Care 1997;42:364-369.
6. Ellis ER, McCauley VB, Mellis C, Sullivan CE. Treatment of alveolar hypoventilation in a six year old girl with intermittent positive pressure ventilation through a nose mask. Am Rev Respir Dis 1987;136:188-191.
7. Nielson DW, Black PG. Mask ventilation in congenital central alveolar hypoventilation syndrome. Pediatr Pulmonol 1990;9:44-46.
8. Padman R, Lawless S, Von Nessen S. Use of BiPAP by nasal mask in the treatment of respiratory insufficiency in pediatric patients: preliminary investigation. Pediatr Pulmonol 1994;17:119-123.
9. Rosen CL, D'Andrea L, Haddad GG. Adult criteria for obstructive sleep apnea do not identify children with serious obstruction. Am Rev Respir Dis 1992;146:1231-1234.
10. Teague WG, Kervin L, Dawadkar V, Scott P. Nasal bi-level positive airway pressure acutely improves ventilation and oxygen saturation in children with upper airway obstruction. Am Rev Respir Dis 1991;143:505A.
11. Piper AJ, Parker S, Torzillo PJ, et al. Nocturnal nasal IPPV stabilizes patients with cystic fibrosis and hypercapnic respiratory failure. Chest 1992;102:846-850.
12. Padman R, Nadkarni VN, Von Nessen S, Goodill J. Noninvasive positive pressure ventilation in end-stage cystic fibrosis: a report of seven cases. Respir Care 1994;39:736-739.
13. Brown RW, Grady EA, Van Laanen CJ, et al. Home use of bi-level positive airway pressure (BiPAP) ventilation for chronic respiratory failure in children (abstract). Am J Respir Crit Care Med 1994;149:A376.
14. Fortenberry JD, Del Toro J, Jefferson LS, et al. Management of pediatric acute hypoxemic respiratory insufficiency with bilevel positive pressure (BiPAP) nasal mask ventilation. Chest 1995;108:1059-1064.
15. Akingbola OA, Servant GM, Custer JR, Palmisano JM. Noninvasive bi-level positive pressure ventilation: management of two pediatric patients. Respir Care 1993;38:1092-1098.

16. Akingbola O, Palmisano J, Servant G, et al. Bi-PAP mask ventilation in pediatric patients with acute respiratory failure (abstract). Crit Care Med 1994;22:A144.
17. Meduri GU, Cook TR, Turner RE, et al. Noninvasive positive pressure ventilation in status asthmaticus. Chest 1996;110:767-774.
18. Teague WG, Lowe E, Dominick J, Lang D. Noninvasive positive pressure ventilation (NPPV) in critically ill children with status asthmaticus. Am J Respir Crit Care Med 1998;157:A542.
19. Kacmarek RM. Characteristics of pressure-targeted ventilators used for noninvasive positive pressure ventilation. Respir Care 1997;42:380-388.
20. Ferguson GT, Gilmartin M. CO_2 rebreathing during BiPAP ventilatory assistance. Am J Respir Crit Care Med 1995;151:1126-1135.

Chapter 10

Problems, Remedies, and Strategies to Optimize the Success of Noninvasive Ventilation

Nicholas S. Hill, MD

Introduction

Over the past 12 years, noninvasive positive pressure ventilation (NPPV) has seen rapidly increasing use in both acute and chronic applications. It has gained acceptance as the ventilator modality of first choice for patients with acute respiratory failure due to exacerbations of chronic obstructive pulmonary disease (COPD) and chronic respiratory failure due to chest wall disorders or neuromuscular diseases.[1] When used appropriately, NPPV should enhance patient comfort and convenience, reduce morbidity by avoiding the complications of invasive ventilation, and decrease the cost of medical care.[2,3] Although it is generally safe and tolerated by most patients, NPPV is not free of adverse side effects or complications, and reported failure rates range from below 10% to more than 40% in published studies.[4] The following discussion reviews the commonly encountered problems associated with NPPV use, provides possible remedies, and suggests ways of optimizing success rates.

Problems Related to the Mask

The most common problems encountered during use of NPPV are related to the mask (or interface) (Table 1). The different types of interfaces used to administer NPPV share some problems, but others depend on mask type. Thus, problems arising with the use of each mask type will be discussed separately.

From *Noninvasive Positive Pressure Ventilation: Principles and Applications,* edited by Nicholas S. Hill. © 2001, Futura Publishing Company, Inc., Armonk, NY.

Table 1
Problems Related to Masks During NPPV

Problem	Incidence	Remedy
Nasal Masks		
Mask discomfort	30–50%	Adjust strap tension, reseat mask, try different mask size or type
Skin rashes	10–20%	Topical steroids or clindamycin, dermatologic consultation
Nasal bridge sores	5–10%	Minimize strap tension, use forehead spacer, artificial skin, switch to different mask type
Nasal obstruction	occasional	Topical decongestants, oronasal mask
Oronasal Masks		
Mask discomfort	30–50%	Minimize strap tension, try different mask sizes, or types
Claustrophobia	10–20%	Reassure, switch to different mask type
Skin rashes, nasal bridge sores	10–20%	Same as for nasal mask
Increased dead space	Depends on mask	Insert foam rubber to reduce dead space Antiasphyxia valve
Aspiration/vomiting	Rare	Quick release strap
Mouthpieces		
Discomfort	Common	Reassure, diminishes with adaptation
Hypersalivation, salivary retention	Common	Reassure, diminishes with adaptation
Aerophagia	Common	Reassure, try simethicone
Pressure sores on lips, gums	Infrequent	Adjust strap tension, consider custom fitting
Orthodontic problems	After prolonged use	Remodel mouthpiece, consult orthodontist
Head straps		
Discomfort	10–30%	Try different strap system
Unstable mask	Common with 2-strap system	Try different mask or strap system

Nasal Masks

Nasal masks are the most commonly used types of noninvasive interfaces for chronic respiratory failure. In the acute setting, oronasal masks have been gaining in popularity. Nasal masks are commercially available in numerous sizes and types, and have high rates of patient acceptance for nocturnal ventilation. The standard nasal mask was initially developed for delivery of nasal continuous positive airway pressure (CPAP) to treat obstructive sleep apnea, but investigators soon learned that it also was an effective means of delivering positive pressure ventilation via the nose, mainly in patients with neuromuscular diseases and kyphoscoliosis.[5,6]

As described in Chapter 1, the standard nasal mask consists of a triangular-shaped clear plastic dome that fits over the nose and is connected to ventilator hosing. A soft rubber or silicon gasket makes contact with the skin and creates an air seal. Alternative nasal masks include nasal "pillows" or "seals" that consist of soft rubber cones that insert directly into the nostrils, newer more compact masks, and custom-fitted nasal masks made of prosthetic materials.

Nasal masks are well tolerated in general, but as shown in Table 1, a number of adverse side effects may occur, particularly when the patient is first adapting to the technique. The most common problem is discomfort at points of skin contact, related to the tension necessary to control air leaks. Air leaking through the mouth is also a very common problem during nasal ventilation and is discussed in detail below. The pattern of discomfort depends on mask type, as might be surmised, with the standard nasal mask applying most pressure to the bridge of the nose and cheeks, and nasal pillows to the inner nares. To minimize discomfort, proper fitting of the mask is key, and the least strap tension that acceptably controls air leaks should be used. The use of commercially available fitting gauges is strongly encouraged, and the smallest mask size that just encompasses the nose is usually the best.

The most common error in administering nasal ventilation is to apply excess tension on the straps in an effort to minimize air leaks. Should this occur, the first step should be to make certain that the mask is not too large. Next, the mask should be lifted entirely away from the face and repositioned to assure proper seating of the gasket. Forehead spacers should also be used and replaced at regular intervals to redistribute pressure away from the nasal bridge. Strap tension should be adjusted so that no fewer than two fingers can be accommodated under the strap. Alternatively, different strap systems such as those that are sewed to caps should be tried, to enhance comfort. In general, masks with more points of attachment are more stable and facilitate elimination of leaks, but they may also contribute to feelings of claustrophobia. Masks with very thin plastic flaps ("bubble" mask, Resmed, San Diego, CA; Comfort flaps, Respironics, Inc., Murrysville, PA) over the rubber seal may also enhance air sealing at lower strap tensions.

Pressure sores occur when excessive pressure is applied for too long, leading to ulceration of the nasal bridge in up to 10% of patients. Should ulceration occur, artificial skin may be applied to the area to afford greater protection, and efforts should be redoubled to minimize strap tension. For acute applications, some clinicians advocate the routine prophylactic use of artificial skin over the nasal bridge. If standard nasal masks cause excessive discomfort or unrelenting ulceration, "gel" masks (Goldseal, Respironics; Phantom, SleepNet Corp., Manchester, NH) that have a gel-filled gasket, or masks with specially molded soft silicone seals (Mirage, Resmed) may bring relief. One gel mask (Blueseal, Respironics) molds to the contour of the face when heated. Alternatively, nasal pillows may be used to eliminate contact with the bridge of the nose and cheeks, but patients may find these just as uncomfortable as standard masks because of pressure in the nares. In this case, alternating between the two mask types may offer a solution. For patients who experience claustrophobic reactions with standard nasal masks, nasal pillows or newer minimasks (Monarch or Simplicity, Respironics) that are more compact and use softer rubber for nasal sealing may be helpful. With the ever expanding variety of nasal masks commercially available, an acceptable mask assembly can almost always be found, and custom fitting is rarely necessary.

Oronasal or Full Face Masks

Oronasal masks cover both the nose and mouth and are preferred by some clinicians for the therapy of acute respiratory failure. This preference is based on the belief that patients with acute respiratory distress are mouth breathers and will tolerate oronasal masks better than nasal masks. In fact there is little evidence to support this view, and success rates of studies using nasal masks for delivery of NPPV to patients with acute respiratory failure compare favorably with those of studies using oronasal masks. In one study on patients with chronic respiratory failure, oronasal masks were more effective at lowering $PaCO_2$ than nasal masks, but were less well tolerated.[7] Oronasal masks are prone to the same local problems as nasal masks (Table 1), with essentially the same remedies.

Compared to nasal masks, oronasal masks may reduce air leaks through the mouth or under the mask, particularly in edentulous patients. On the other hand, nasal masks permit easier speech and eating during use. Oronasal masks, like nasal masks, cause discomfort at areas of skin contact as well as ulcerations at the bridge of the nose (Figure 1). Oronasal masks with soft silicone gaskets (such as the Mirage, Resmed) appear to be less likely to cause such sores. Claustrophobic reactions are more often encountered with oronasal masks than with nasal masks, because of the greater bulk. Also, although air leaks through the mouth may be reduced, leaks between the mask gasket and chin may be a persistent problem.

Another risk associated with the use of oronasal masks is aspiration during emesis because of vomitus retained in the mask. This concern has led to the recommendation that a nasogastric tube be used routinely with oronasal ventilation.[8] However, because the complica-

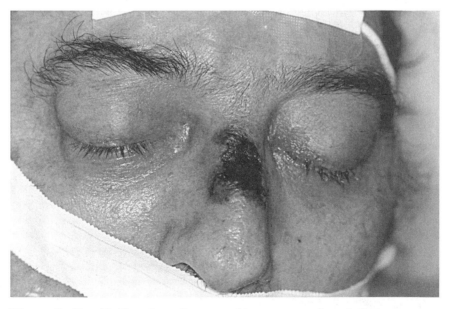

Figure 1. Nasal bridge ulceration caused by an oronasal mask that was excessively tightened. Optimal fitting of the mask, use of the minimal strap tension that controls air leaks, and routine application of artificial skin to the nasal bridge reduce the occurrence of this complication. (With permission from Hill NS. Complications of noninvasive positive pressure ventilation. Respir Care 1997;42:432–442.)

tion of aspiration is unusual if appropriate patients are chosen, nasogastric tubes are unnecessary unless patients have other indications such as nausea and vomiting or abdominal pain with distention. Oronasal masks have more dead space than nasal masks, and because they cover both the nose and mouth, asphyxiation is a concern in the event of ventilator failure if the patient is incapable of removing the mask. For this reason, some clinicians fill masks with foam rubber to reduce dead space, and masks specifically designed for NPPV have so-called "anti-asphyxia valves" to prevent rebreathing if the ventilator fails. As with nasal masks, most patients can successfully tolerate one of the commercially available oronasal masks, and the most important ways to enhance acceptance are to optimize fit and avoid excessive strap tension.

Mouthpiece Ventilation

Lipseals, mouthpieces, and custom-fitted orthodontic devices have been used less widely than nasal or oronasal masks, and fewer descriptions have been published. Nonetheless, successful application of NPPV via mouthpiece has been reported in a large number of patients with neuromuscular disease.[9] Common problems associated with lipseal ventilation include discomfort caused by foreign material in the mouth and pressure from the lipseal, aerophagia, hypersalivation, and difficulty swallowing with retention of saliva. Pressure sores occur on the cheeks or gums when lipseals are strapped on too tightly. Air leakage around the lipseal or through the nose may impair efficacy, sometimes necessitating insertion of nasal plugs or use of nose clips. Growth of a mustache and/or beard can interfere with air sealing during lipseal use, contributing to hypoventilation. Most of these problems can be addressed by fitting adjustments and allowing time for adaptation, but in the author's experience, commercially available mouthpieces and lipseals are less well tolerated by patients than nasal masks.

Some centers have reported excellent results with custom-made mouthpieces fitted by an oral prosthetist.[9] In addition to the above-listed adverse effects, these custom-made devices have caused occasional allergic reactions to the prosthetic materials and dental deformation after years of use. In one study on 257 mouthpiece users with neuromuscular disease, 11 deaths occurred, some when the mouthpiece accidentally fell out in patients who were dependent on mechanical ventilation.[9] Therefore, adequate monitoring and alarms for such patients are advisable. These prosthetic devices have some advantages over nasal and oronasal masks, however, including reduced air leakage in some patients. Some patients also find custom-made mouthpieces more tolerable because straps may be unnecessary, and there is less foreign material in contact with the face.

Headgear

The strap system designed to hold the mask in place may contribute to patient discomfort. Some straps are thin with relatively rough surfaces. Others slide during use, contributing to mask instability and air leaks, and sometimes abrading the cheeks or ears. Most masks come with predesigned strap systems, and options to modify them may be limited. Nonetheless, communication with the manufacturer may yield suggestions for modification or advice on how to contact sources of custom-made straps. In general, strap stability is enhanced by more points of contact with the mask or by sewing the strap to a cap.

Problems Related to Air Pressure and Flow

Discomfort related to air pressure is very commonly encountered during initiation of NPPV, both in the acute and chronic settings (Table 2). Air pressure in the nose and sinuses may cause sinus or ear pain, burning, or coldness. For this reason, NPPV should be initiated with relatively low peak inspiratory pressures (8–12 cm H_2O). Pressures can then be gradually titrated upward with close attention to patient response. In the acute setting, pressures are adjusted upward more rapidly so that respiratory distress is alleviated, but in the chronic setting, clinicians should be patient with pressure increases, taking up to 1 or 2 months or more before reaching optimal pressures. Overly aggressive pressure increases may greatly interfere with patient adaptation, particularly if the desire is to have the patient sleeping during NPPV use.

Another frequent problem related to air pressure is gastric insufflation, reported in up to 50% of patients using NPPV.[10] Most patients are aware of some gastric distension and an increase in flatulence or eructation, particularly in the morning if they have been using NPPV overnight. Thankfully, this is rarely severe enough to interfere with therapy. This may be because the lower esophageal sphincter pressure is greater than 20 cm H_2O most of the time and may rise to as high as 60 mm Hg,[11] far exceeding typical inspiratory pressures during NPPV.

Table 2
Problems Related to Air Pressure and Flow

Problem	Incidence	Remedy
Pressure		
Discomfort	20–50%	Reduce inspiratory pressure
Ear, sinus pain	10–20%	Reduce inspiratory pressure
Gastric insufflation	30–40%	Reduce pressure, simethacone, gastric suction if ventilation impaired
Pneumothorax	Rare	Avoid excessive inflation pressures, consider thoracostomy tube drainage
Flow		
Nasal/oral congestion	50%	Topical steroids, decongestants, antihistamine/decongestant combinations
Nasal/oral dryness	30–50%	Nasal saline, humidification, control of air leaks
Eye irritation	33%	Reduce air leakage, eye emollients, try adjusting strap tension, different mask

However, lower esophageal sphincter pressure falls during swallowing and in response to acute illness and many medications. Thus, gastric insufflation occurs not infrequently during NPPV and may be exacerbated by aerophagia. In fact, the only patient that the author has encountered who found gastric distension intolerable during NPPV failed to improve after a gastric tube and eventual tracheostomy, suggesting that her symptoms were at least in part due to aerophagia.

With regard to therapy, less symptomatic patients may respond to reductions in inspiratory pressure or defoaming agents like simethicone, or they may simply tolerate the symptom without treatment. More symptomatic patients may be difficult to treat. Minimization of inspiratory pressure and experimenting with positional eructation may help. As mentioned above, aerophagia may be contributing but is a difficult behavior to eradicate. Placement of gastric tubes should be avoided unless all other measures have failed, and the gastric distension is intolerable or is interfering with ventilation.

More serious consequences of excessive inflation pressure such as pulmonary barotrauma occur rarely during NPPV because inflation pressures are usually much lower than those used during invasive ventilation (<25 cm H_2O). The author has encountered two patients with barotrauma, brother and sister, who developed recurrent pneumo-thoraces while receiving NPPV, both after inflation pressures had been increased from 14 cm H_2O to 16 cm H_2O in one and 18 cm H_2O to 20 cm H_2O in the other.[4] Both had apical blebs that likely contributed to the problem. One patient required tube evacuation and sclerosis, and the other required open pleurodesis. Although no studies have formally studied the possibility, ventilator-induced lung injury[12] would not be anticipated with NPPV, because plateau pressures rarely exceed 20 cm H_2O.

Nasal congestion and dryness are also common complaints during NPPV, sometimes occurring in the same patient. Mouth drooling and dryness are also common, the latter usually associated with air leaking through the mouth. Nasal congestion usually responds to nasal steroids or antihistamine/decongestant combinations. Nasal congestion associated with upper respiratory infections probably interferes with the efficacy of NPPV, and topical vasoconstrictors may be useful temporarily during such periods. Nasal dryness, often associated with a sensation of cold or burning, may respond to the use of topical saline or emollient sprays. Oral dryness may respond to measures aimed at reducing mouth leaks, such as chin straps. If dryness fails to respond to these measures, though, a humidifier should be added to the breathing circuit. The high flow of cool, dry air through the nose during mouth leakage has been shown to increase nasal resistance, and this is lessened by warmed, humidified air.[13]

When "bilevel" type pressure-limited ventilators are used, only pass-over humidifiers should be used. Heat and moisture exchangers and bubble-through humidifiers should be avoided because of increases in ventilator circuit resistance and lowered inspiratory pressures associated with their use. When nasal dryness becomes severe, epistaxis may occur during use of nasal ventilation. This is treated with standard local measures and humidification, and nasal saline or lubricating jelly gently applied to the internal surface of the affected nares may prevent further episodes. Petroleum jelly is to be avoided because of the possibility of aspiration.

Eye irritation is another adverse effect of air flow associated with the use of standard nasal or oronasal masks that has been reported in up to a third of patients.[10] It is caused by leakage of air under the mask on the sides of the nose lateral to the nasal bridge, where effective air sealing is difficult. This is occasionally caused by excessive tightening of mask straps and may respond to loosening, or use of soothing eye drops. More often, however, the problem is related to an ill-fitting mask and an alternative mask must be used to correct the problem.

Alternatives include the use of comfort flaps, switching to a bubble mask, or trying nasal pillows.

Major Complications (Table 3)

Complications that lead to significant medical morbidity are unusual with NPPV if patients are carefully selected, and skilled, experienced personnel apply the modality. The most common significant complication among reported series on acute respiratory failure has been aspiration pneumonia, reported in one of 20 patients in one series.[8] This is an inherent risk because of the lack of airway protection afforded by NPPV and the reliance on the patient's airway protective mechanisms. In the author's experience, this is a very infrequent complication, seen most often in patients who are reluctant or decline to undergo endotracheal intubation and may have some impairment of airway protective mechanisms, but nonetheless desire a trial with noninvasive ventilation. The risks of this complication are minimized by exclusion of patients with significant impairment of upper airway protective mechanisms, or placement of a nasogastric tube in those predisposed to vomiting by virtue of gross gastric distension, an ileus or bowel obstruction.

Other major complications in the acute setting include mucus plugging, hypoxemia,[14] and respiratory arrest during NPPV use. Mucus plug-

Table 3
Major Complications

Problem	Occurrence	Remedy
Aspiration	5%	Careful patient selection, gastric drainage when appropriate
Mucus plugging	Infrequent	Careful patient selection, adequate rehydration, cough assistance, respiratory treatments
Severe hypoxemia	*	Proper patient selection, high flow O_2, increased expiratory pressure
Hypotension	Infrequent	Proper patient selection, adequate hydration, lower inspiratory pressures

*Depends on etiology of respiratory failure.

ging can be minimized if patients are kept well hydrated and cough assistive techniques are applied, particularly in those with neuromuscular disease and reduced peak expiratory flows.[15] Respiratory treatments with aerosolized bronchodilators may also help with secretion removal, and these may be administered directly into the ventilator tubing without interrupting NPPV.[16]

Hypoxemia during NPPV use may occur as a consequence of mucus plugging, but adequate oxygenation is usually not difficult to achieve in patients with hypercapnic respiratory failure. With bilevel ventilators, oxygen tubing is connected directly to the mask or to a "T" valve in the ventilator circuit, and flow rate is titrated upward until an adequate oxygen saturation has been achieved. Flow rates as high as 10–15 L/min are sometimes used without obvious untoward effects. Rates as high as 40 L/min have been reported,[14] although it has not been established how effective such high flow rates are or whether triggering and cycling of the ventilator are adversely affected. Assuring adequate oxygenation is more difficult in patients who fail to cooperate in keeping the mask on or in those with hypoxemic respiratory failure (i.e., acute pneumonia or adult respiratory distress syndrome). Although NPPV has been reported to be as efficacious in oxygenating these patients as invasive ventilation,[17] successful NPPV administration in these patients can be challenging. In such patients, the use of ventilators with oxygen blenders that provide accurate FiO_2s up to 100% is recommended. In addition, increases in expiratory pressure may be helpful to reduce FiO_2 requirements. Of course, increases in inspiratory pressure must match the increased expiratory pressure if pressure support is to be maintained, and this may lead to intolerance if pressures are excessive.

Hypotension is an infrequent problem during NPPV if patients are properly selected. Pressures used during NPPV are relatively low, and frankly hypotensive patients are usually excluded as NPPV candidates. On the other hand, patients with low intravascular fluid volume may develop hypotension even with low pressure CPAP or NPPV. Therefore, the clinician must make certain that fluid volume is adequate if hypotension occurs during NPPV use. If hypotension occurs in a patient with a COPD exacerbation, the possibility of auto-PEEP (positive end-expiratory pressure) should also be considered. The patient should be coached to adopt a slower breathing pattern, and shortening the rise time and maximal inspiratory duration (in ventilators that have this capability) may allow more time for exhalation. If hypotension and evidence of organ hypoperfusion persist despite these measures, intravenous pressors can be initiated, but in patients with evidence of organ hypoperfusion, prompt intubation and controlled breathing are usually recommended to minimize oxygen consumption by the breathing muscles.

CPAP has been shown to favorably affect hemodynamics in patients with cardiac failure, but this depends on the relative effects of the increased intrathoracic pressure on preload versus afterload.[18] By increasing intrathoracic pressure in patients with high preload and afterload, CPAP can lower preload by decreasing venous return, and afterload by reducing the pressure gradient between the thorax and peripheral vasculature. However, if preload is lowered excessively by increases in intrathoracic pressure, organ perfusion could be adversely affected. This could explain a recent observation on patients with acute pulmonary edema randomized to receive CPAP (10 cm H_2O) or bilevel positive airway pressure (BiPAP) (15 cm H_2O inspiratory and 5 cm H_2O expiratory pressures). In this study,[19] patients using BiPAP had a more rapid improvement in ventilation and respiratory rate than patients on CPAP, but they also had a more abrupt decrease in blood pressure, associated with a higher rate of nontransmural myocardial infarctions. Although some of the BiPAP patients may have been in the process of infarcting before admission, this finding underscores the need for caution in selecting initial pressures and close monitoring of hemodynamics in patients using NPPV at risk for cardiac ischemia.

Other major problems and complications include progressive respiratory failure unresponsive to NPPV leading to intubation, and cardiorespiratory arrest during use. Obviously, immediate intubation is warranted in patients suffering a respiratory or cardiac arrest during NPPV use. This usually reflects a major cardiopulmonary crisis such as central airway obstruction, "flash" pulmonary edema, arrhythmia, or circulatory failure. This underscores the need to adequately monitor patients undergoing NPPV for acute respiratory failure. Patients who are at risk for respiratory arrest if the mask becomes disconnected must be managed in a closely monitored setting such as an intensive care unit (ICU) or step-down unit. Only after they have stabilized and are capable of breathing free of the ventilator for 20–30 minutes at a time should transfer to a regular floor be contemplated. In countries where respiratory intensive care beds are few, ICU monitoring is preferred for potentially unstable patients. A recent randomized controlled trial from England demonstrated that less acutely ill COPD patients can be successfully managed using NPPV on a respiratory general ward, as long as pH was > 7.30.[20]

Strategies to minimize NPPV failure are discussed below, but measures should also be undertaken to avoid cardiopulmonary arrest during NPPV. Patients should be watched closely during the first few hours of use. If clear indications of a favorable response are not apparent, such as decreased $PaCO_2$, respiratory rate, or sternocleidomastoid muscle activity, then the patient should be intubated if ventilatory assistance is still warranted. Persisting with NPPV for more than a few hours in patients who remain intolerant and show no signs of improving is not only counterproductive, but may be harmful to the patient who is likely to become more and more fatigued and who may arrest. This may explain why there was a trend for increased mortality among patients treated with NPPV in an emergency department where the average delay before intubation in patients who failed was greater than 24 hours.[21]

Reasons for NPPV Failure and Strategies to Optimize Success (Table 4)

Patient Selection

One of the most important aspects of successful implementation of NPPV is selection of appropriate patients. This topic is discussed in detail in the previous chapters dealing with the specific etiology of respiratory failure, and will be discussed only in general terms here. Patient choice is a major determinant of the likelihood that a patient will tolerate NPPV or be successfully ventilated. Thus, widely accepted selection guidelines should be followed to optimize the chances of success. Of course, patients who are mildly ill and not really in need of ventilatory assistance will likely avoid intubation whether they go on NPPV or not. These patients might be counted as "successes" when, in fact, they indicate a failure to appropriately use resources. Thus, patients should be screened using clinical and blood gas criteria to ascertain that they are sick enough to require ventilatory assistance. On the other hand, it is clear that patients who are allowed to deteriorate before NPPV is initiated or who are too sick (as determined by APACHE scores) fare less well on NPPV.[22] Thus, there is a "window of opportunity" for optimal application of NPPV, when patients are ill enough to require ventilatory assistance, but not so ill as to make success unlikely.

At least as important as screening out patients who do not really need ventilatory assistance is excluding those who are at higher risk if NPPV is used. This is detailed in Chapters 2-7, but in general, the ideal candidate breathes spontaneously, has no medical instability

Table 4
Reasons for Failure to Ventilate

Reason	Remedy
Inappropriate patient	Proper patient selection
Failure to tolerate mask	Optimize size, fit, try different types
Nasal obstruction	Nasal decongestant
Ventilator intolerance	Careful titration of inspiratory pressure
Patient-ventilation synchrony	Adjust rise time, trigger sensitivity, inspiratory duration
Agitation, uncooperativeness	Assure comfort, reassure, encourage, judicious sedation
Inadequate ventilator pressures	Increased pressure support or tidal volume (inspiratory-expiratory pressure difference)
Patient noncompliance	Encourage increased use
Secretion retention	Cough assistance devices, adequate humidification, hydration, N-acetyl cysteine
Air leaks	Avoid overventilation, try chin straps, optimize mask fit, switch to different mask
Rebreathing	Expiratory pressure ≥ 4 cm H_2O, minimize mask dead space, non-rebreathing valves
Clinician inexperience	Well-trained, motivated, and experienced staff

other than respiratory, is able to protect the upper airway and cooperate, and can accommodate a well-fitting interface. Particularly for the chronic setting, but to a certain extent in the acute setting, the ideal patient should be motivated and have a reasonable capacity to comprehend instructions. As discussed in more detail below, the failure to observe these guidelines leads to inclusion of patients who will have a great deal of difficulty tolerating or ventilating adequately with NPPV.

Patient Characteristics

Patient characteristics such as mechanical properties of the respiratory system and underlying diagnosis also have an influence on outcome. In the acute setting, evidence from a number of groups suggests that patients with pneumonia fare less well, perhaps because of the likelihood of problems with secretion clearance, whereas those with uncomplicated COPD do quite well.[22] Patients with markedly altered respiratory mechanics and gas exchange such those with low lung compliance and severe hypoxemia due to pulmonary fibrosis also may be harder to support noninvasively than invasively. In fact, no series has reported successful use of NPPV in these patients. On the other hand, patients with low compliance due to chest wall deformities, or high resistance due to COPD may respond very well to NPPV.

Failure to Tolerate NPPV

Mask Intolerance

In both acute and chronic settings, a substantial minority of appropriately selected patients will be unable to tolerate NPPV. Success rates are quite high in patients with chronic respiratory failure due to neuromuscular or chest wall disorders (averaging 80–90%) and substantially lower in patients with severe stable COPD (perhaps 50%).[23] In the acute setting, reported success rates have varied from 58–93%.[2,3,8] In both acute and chronic settings, mask intolerance is a very important cause for failure. With patience, ingenuity and persistence, the experienced practitioner should still be able to achieve success in many patients having difficulty with mask tolerance, but at the expense of additional time. Proper fit of the mask and optimization of the strap system should first be assured. Different mask sizes and types should be tried if the patient is unable to tolerate the initial choice. Some patients tolerate oronasal masks when nasal masks fail, and vice versa.

Nasal obstruction may cause failure of NPPV in some patients, either due to congestion, polyps, septal deviation, or some other anatomic abnormality. A topical decongestant may be quite effective in ameliorating it. Oversized oral masks and excessive strap tension should be avoided. Attaching a bag that contains various mask types and sizes to ventilators used for NPPV assures ready availability when addressing mask tolerance problems. Other manipulations, such as adjusting body or head position may occasionally help.

Ventilator Intolerance

Excessively rapid increases in pressure lead to intolerance by causing pain in the sinuses or ears and frightening patients, contributing to agitation. Setting of pressures should be a gradual process carried out at the bedside while paying close attention to patient response.

Particularly in the acute setting, pressures must be advanced rapidly enough to diminish work of breathing and afford relief of respiratory distress. However, this must be balanced against the likelihood of intolerable discomfort if the clinician focuses exclusively on alleviation of breathing effort. It should be borne in mind that for many patients, a partial reduction in breathing effort is sufficient to restore a balance in the supply/demand relationship of breathing work. Accordingly, selection of pressures can be seen as a compromise between the desire to reduce the work of breathing as much as possible and the need to minimize discomfort.

Patient-Ventilator Asynchrony

Another contributor to ventilator intolerance is difficulty with patient-ventilator synchrony. As discussed below, this may also contribute to failure to ventilate, but it is an important element in optimization of patient comfort. An insufficiently sensitive ventilator trigger may lead to failure to lower inspiratory effort, whereas an overly sensitive trigger may cause auto-cycling. Likewise, in ventilators that have an adjustable "rise time," an excessively rapid inspiratory flow may contribute to discomfort in neuromuscular patients, whereas patients with COPD often prefer a high inspiratory flow rate and may become uncomfortable if rise time is too long.[24] Further, as discussed earlier, pressure support modes may have difficulty cycling in synchrony with termination of the patient's inspiratory effort in the presence of air leaks or in patients with COPD. Patients with COPD often have high initial inspiratory flow rates and short inspiratory times, predisposing to a delay in ventilator cycling to expiration.[25] In these situations, adjustments in inspiratory and/or expiratory sensitivity (with the Knightstar 335, Mallinckrodt, St. Louis, MO) or limiting inspiratory duration (with the VPAP STA, Resmed or Vision, Respironics) may help. Alternatively, switching to a pressure assist/control mode so that cycling occurs via a timer,[26] and optimization of rise time (with the VPAP STA or Quantum, Respironics) may enable patients to tolerate the ventilator. If the ventilator being used does not offer these adjustments in an intolerant patient, switching to one that does may be useful. Other ventilator adjustments, such as adding PEEP in patients with presumed auto-PEEP, or silencing alarms when initiating NPPV, may facilitate acceptance. Finally, agitation is a major cause of asynchrony, rendering patients unable to coordinate their breathing with the ventilator, as discussed below.

Agitation

Agitation and inability to cooperate are other common reasons for intolerance. Of course, patients who have obvious agitation and are pulling off oxygen masks and removing intravenous tubing should not be treated with NPPV at all. However, some patients become agitated and uncooperative after intitiation, perhaps because of discomfort or fear related to the procedure, and sometimes because of progression of their disease. In any case, this development threatens the success of NPPV. In response, the clinician must do a prompt bedside assessment to determine whether agitation is related to discomfort and whether adjustments in mask fitting or ventilator settings can restore patient acceptance. If these appear to be optimized, communication with the patient may be helpful. The patient should be reassured and encouraged not to give up easily. Coaching of breathing pattern and the suggestion that patients "try to let the machine breathe for them" may be helpful. Also, a reminder to the patient that, if NPPV is successful, intubation will be unnecessary, may serve as a strong motivator. In the acute setting, judicious use of sedation may aid in acceptance. In the chronic setting, use of sedation is discouraged, but it should be pointed out to patients that adapting to NPPV is not unlike learning to master a musical instrument. Frequent practice sessions are required, and months may pass before patients become "expert" at the technique.

Despite all these efforts, some patients (perhaps 10–15%) remain unable to tolerate the sensation of a foreign object on the face or air flow in the nose or mouth. These patients may suffer from claustrophobia or may be very anxious or sensitive to objects strapped to the face. In the acute setting, these patients may need expedient intubation if respiratory failure persists. Most investigators agree that if tolerance of NPPV is not achieved within a maximum of 2–3 hours, as demonstrated by a reduction in respiratory rate and (in hypercapnic patients) a decline in $PaCO_2$, prompt intubation should be carried out if the patient still requires ventilatory assistance. In the chronic setting, other forms of noninvasive ventilation such as negative pressure or abdominal ventilation may be tried before resorting to tracheostomy.[27]

Failure to Ventilate Adequately

Many studies have distinguished between failure to tolerate and failure to ventilate as causes of unsuccessful application of NPPV.

Obviously, there is considerable overlap between these categories; patients who are unable to tolerate NPPV are unlikely to receive sufficient ventilatory assistance. On the other hand, it is often possible to identify patients who fail primarily because of their intolerance of the equipment as opposed to those who can tolerate the mask and ventilator settings and simply fail to improve their ventilation. The inability to adequately assist ventilation has varied considerably between reported studies, causing failure of NPPV in from 7% to approximately 50% of patients. This undoubtedly reflects differences in the selection criteria used between studies, as well as variable skills and experience between centers. The major contributors to failure to ventilate are listed in Table 4 and are discussed in more detail in the following section.

Inadequate Ventilator Settings and Patient Noncompliance

In the acute setting, failure to improve ventilation may be related to inadequate inspiratory assistance, and may respond to increases in inspiratory pressure. It should be borne in mind that, during pressure-limited ventilation, inspiratory assistance is determined more by the difference between the inspiratory and expiratory pressures than the inspiratory pressure per se. Thus, an increase in expiratory pressure to a high level necessitates equal increases in inspiratory pressure if the level of inspiratory assistance is to be maintained. Of course, excessive increases in pressure in an effort to improve ventilation may cause ventilator intolerance, as discussed above, and sometimes, it is impossible to find pressures that augment ventilation and are still tolerable to the patient. It is also sometimes difficult to achieve adequate ventilatory assistance in the acute setting because the patient keeps removing the mask and refuses to use it for a sufficient period of time to gain benefit. Beyond encouragement, judicious sedation, and gentle restraints, measures to improve compliance in these patients are limited; some patients will require intubation if blood gases remain poor or worsen.

In the chronic setting, failure to adequately ventilate may also be caused by insufficient inflation pressures or delivered tidal volumes, or inadequate duration of use by the patient. Some patients experience great difficulty adapting to NPPV and are able to use it for only 1 or 2 hours at bedtime. This is usually inadequate to bring about sustained improvements in alveolar ventilation. In this situation, visits by a home respiratory therapist can be very helpful to evaluate mask fit and ventilator settings, and to make sure the patient is using the equipment correctly. The therapist tries alternative interfaces, reassures the patient that adaptation may be a lengthy process, and encourages the patient to gradually extend periods of nocturnal use. Some improvements in symptoms and gas exchange (as measured by blood gases or daytime oximetry and end-tidal $PaCO_2$) can be anticipated once the patient is using the device for at least 4–6 hours nightly. If no improvements are apparent, the patient should be encouraged to continue extending periods of use, and the ventilator timer should be checked to confirm reported hours of use.

Inspiratory pressures or delivered tidal volumes should also be gradually increased as tolerated. In general, substantial improvements in daytime gas exchange are not seen unless the patient is using inspiratory pressures of at least 12 cm H_2O for at least 4–6 hours nightly, depending on mechanical properties of the respiratory system, of course. Because patients often overestimate the number of hours of use,[23] it is useful to check actual recorded hours of use as recorded by the clock on the home ventilator. Some ventilators even record number of hours above a certain pressure to make certain that the clock is not merely measuring the number of hours the machine is turned on. If adequate compliance is documented, and there is no improvement even after the patient is sleeping through the night using inspiratory pressures > 12 cm H_2O, the patient should be monitored nocturnally using a multichannel recorder. Evidence should be sought of persisting hypoventilation, apneas, or excessive air leaks. Hypoventilation may still respond to further increases in inflation pressure or duration of ventilation, but if persisting obstructive apneas and hypopneas are observed, expiratory pressure should be adjusted to eliminate them by splinting open the upper airway at the initiation of inspiration. Repeat nocturnal monitoring is indicated to ascertain whether the PEEP level is adequate. Nocturnal monitoring is also useful when patients who had previously been stabilized using NPPV experience recurrent symptoms and worsening hypoventilation. These patients often respond to increases in inspiratory pressure and/or greater duration of ventilator use.

Secretion Retention

NPPV is contraindicated in patients with excessive secretions or who are unable to adequately protect their airway because of impaired swallowing or cough impairment. However, this is a relative contraindication, and deciding when secretions are excessive or the ability to protect the upper airway is too impaired is a matter of clinical judgment. Many patients begun on NPPV have the need to expectorate frequently, and may have some weakening of the cough reflex or swallowing dysfunction. Because NPPV sacrifices control of the airway, other measures besides endotracheal suctioning must be applied to these patients. Use of a nasal, rather than oronasal, mask may facilitate expectoration in some patients. In COPD patients, adequate hydration and frequent respiratory treatments may be useful. In patients with weakened expiratory muscles or severe restriction, who have reduced peak cough flows, measures aimed at assisting coughing may help in secretion removal.[15] These include manually assisted coughing, during which a midepigastric thrust using the palm of the assistant's hand is timed with coughing, or mechanical devices (see Chapter 1). One such device, the cough In-Exsufflator (JH Emerson, Cambridge, MA), inflates the lungs with positive pressure (30–40 cm H_2O) via a face mask and rapidly switches to a comparable negative pressure, simulating a cough maneuver. Other measures include chest physiotherapy or N-acetyl cysteine, in some patients. However, when these measures fail or when swallowing is severely impaired, conversion to invasive ventilation is usually necessary. This potential complication underscores the importance of carefully screening NPPV candidates for the ability to protect the airway.

Air Leaks

Because of the lack of an airtight connection to the lower airways, NPPV is inherently leaky. Achieving a leak-free air seal between mask and face is nearly impossible, but mask leaks can usually be reduced to acceptable levels. The greater challenge is to control leaks and achieve adequate alveolar ventilation while relying on upper airway structures that permit air to take a number of routes besides entry into the lungs. These alternative routes include mouth leaks during nasal ventilation, nasal leaks during mouthpiece ventilation, and esophageal insufflation during any form of NPPV. Awake, cooperative subjects can usually be coached to keep their mouths closed and coordinate their breathing with the ventilator so that it assists their breathing, but this is nearly impossible in agitated, uncooperative patients. However, when patients become inattentive or fall asleep, the success of NPPV depends on the continued flow of air through the upper airway into the lungs.

It is not entirely clear how inattentive or sleeping subjects permit air to enter their lungs when it is forced in from a mask, or how the respiratory center modifies its output in response to NPPV. Mechanisms by which this is achieved are not fully understood, but direct visualization of the upper airway during NPPV in awake and sleeping has provided some insight.[28,29] In these studies, glottic aperture was an important determinant of air entry into the lungs. As compared to the awake state, this aperture narrowed slightly during stages 1 and 2 sleep, and widened during deeper stages of sleep. In addition, increases in delivered tidal volume and resulting reductions in end-tidal PCO_2 correlated with narrowing of the aperture, reducing the proportion of air entering the lungs. Thus, glottic narrowing is one mechanism contributing to air leaking through the mouth. However, other mechanisms may be important, such as positioning of the soft palate and mandible.

Some leaking of air, either around the mask, through the mouth with nasal ventilation, or through the nose with mouth ventilation, is inevitable during NPPV. Air leakage through the mouth has been observed during the majority of sleep in 7 patients with kyphoscoliosis who were receiving volume-limited nasal ventilation.[30] An association was detected between leakage and sleep fragmentation, characterized by lightening of sleep stage and brief arousals. These arousals were most apt to occur during brief oxygen desaturations associated with the leakage, so hypoxemia was presumed to be the mechanism for the arousals. Another investigation on 6 patients using pressure-limited ventilation, most with neuromuscular disease, also found leakage during the majority of sleep.[31] The prevalence of leakage was associated with sleep stage, occurring less often (62%) during stage 1 sleep and most often (100%) during slow wave sleep (SWS, stages 3 and 4). This latter study also found an association between air leakage and arousals.

These studies demonstrate that although air leakage is highly prevalent during use of NPPV, it does not always impair efficacy. Ventilation and oxygenation may be adequately supported despite prolonged periods of leakage, depending on the ventilator used and adaptive mechanisms of the patient. Sleep fragmentation due to leak-associated arousals appears to be the major adverse consequence of leakage in most patients.[31] However, when it is apparent that leakage is compromising ventilatory assistance, switching to a ventilator that has good leak-compensating capabilities (such as a portable pressure support ventilator) may help. In addition, adding chin straps may reduce leakage through the mouth during nasal ventilation. Alternatively, switching to an oronasal mask or mouthpiece may ameliorate the problem, although leaking can occur with any mask type. Increasing insufflation pressure or tidal volume to compensate for leaks may not always be the best strategy, because this could increase mask pressure or lead to glottic narrowing and exacerbate the leakage. Firm recommendations on the best way to deal with air leaks await more studies on compensatory upper airway mechanisms and the consequences of leakage.

Rebreathing

Rebreathing may occur during use of portable pressure support (bilevel) ventilators because of the single lumen ventilator circuit that serves as both inspiratory and expiratory tubing. These ventilators are designed to function with a continuous leak through an exhalation port located in the mask or in the distal end of the ventilator tubing. This port is usually fixed and serves as the exhaust port for CO_2 exhaled into the circuit. The phenomenon of rebreathing with these ventilators was first described during use of the BiPAP S/T (Respironics, Inc.).[32] Use of the the Whisper Swivel Connector (Respironics, Inc) exhalation valve was shown to induce substantial rebreathing when expiratory pressures on the BiPAP were low (<4 cm H_2O). The rebreathing was enough to prevent reduction in CO_2 among patients during a brief daytime trial. The problem was ameliorated by maintaining adequate bias flows with expiratory pressures > 4 cm H_2O or by using other exhalation valves that prevent rebreathing, such as the Plateau or NRB (non-rebreathing) valves (Respironics, Inc.).

Lofaso et al.[33] also noted rebreathing using the BiPAP ventilator that was eliminated by use of non-rebreathing valves, but these valves increased expiratory resistance. Although the phenomenon of rebreathing has been well-described in laboratory settings, its importance has not been established in well-designed clinical studies. A recent preliminary evaluation on 6 long-term users of NPPV using nasal BiPAP nocturnally found that switching to a Plateau non-rebreathing valve from a Whisper Swivel Connector had no effect on daytime or nocturnal gas exchange or symptoms.[33] Also, because of the commonness of leaking around the mask or through the mouth, much of the exhaled CO_2 never entered the exhalation tubing. The clinical importance of rebreathing has not been evaluated in the acute setting or during use of an oronasal mask. It is likely that rebreathing is greater during oronasal than nasal ventilation because CO_2 exhaled through the mouth may be rebreathed as well. On the other hand, it has not been shown that a small amount of rebreathing or lowering $PaCO_2$ to a slightly higher level than would be the case with a non-rebreathing valve is deleterious in any way. If the clinician wishes to minimize the amount of rebreathing, maintenance of an expiratory pressure of 4 cm H_2O or greater will assure enough bias flow to reduce rebreathing, and use of non-rebreathing or Plateau valves or ventilators with separate inspiratory and expiratory tubing will eliminate the problem.

Clinician Inexperience and Impatience

Thus far, we have discussed failure of NPPV caused by equipment or patient-related factors. However, the importance of communication between caregivers and patients is greater than with invasive ventilation and its role in eventual success should not be underestimated. In the acute setting, staff that convey a sense of confidence and competence are far more apt to gain patient trust and cooperation than those who seem incompetent and pessimistic. Clinicians who are willing to spend extra time and effort assuring that patient comfort and ventilator settings are optimized are much more often rewarded with success. Caregivers must coach patients to adapt their breathing patterns to the ventilator and reassure them so that they relax sufficiently to allow the ventilator to assist their breathing. Often in the acute setting, patients are in a state of near panic when NPPV is begun, and the ability to calm them quickly is a skill that comes only with experience. In addition, caregivers must be patient and willing to try different masks and ventilator settings. Giving up too easily contributes to higher failure rates. Identifying a dedicated team of therapists and nurses for administration of NPPV and ensuring that their skills are updated at regular intervals help to assure that success rates are optimized. Of course, staffing must be adequate if therapists and nurses are to have sufficient time to administer NPPV.

In the outpatient setting, there is less urgency in making sure patients are adapted to NPPV, but the need for communication between caregivers and patients is just as great. Patients and their caregivers must be thoroughly trained in the application and maintenance of equipment as well as in dealing with potential problems. Experienced clinicians use aides like teaching mirrors or marked headgear, when appropriate, to facilitate the attachment of masks. In addition, they make periodic home visits and frequent phone calls to detect and address problems before they lead to patient intolerance.

Avoiding Complications

Knowledge of potential problems and their remedies is essential for the successful management of NPPV, but ideally, problems and complications should be anticipated and avoided. Patients are selected using the guidelines discussed previously, and poor candidates for NPPV are avoided. Because so many adverse effects are attributable to the mask, special attention should be paid to mask selection and fitting, as well as headgear tension. Routine use of artificial skin over the bridge of the nose is advisable with both standard nasal and orona- sal masks. The skilled practitioner watches patient response closely, observing both verbal and nonverbal indicators of comfort and respira- tory distress. Ventilator pressures are adjusted promptly, but excessive pressures are avoided. Patients are observed for excessive air leaks or asynchrony with the ventilator, and occasional arterial blood gases are obtained to monitor ventilation. As clinicians gain experience and skill with the management of NPPV, amelioration of problems becomes easier and success rates improve. However, even the most experienced clinicians encounter a minority of patients who are intolerant of the mask or unable to coordinate their breathing with the ventilator, and who will fail to adapt, in perhaps 20–30% of cases.

Summary and Conclusions

NPPV is safe and has few major complications when used in appro- priately selected patients. The most frequently encountered adverse effects are related to the mask and air pressure and flow. These include discomfort, pressure sores on the nasal bridge, dryness and congestion, and pain and burning in the nasal passages and sinuses, depending on the type of interface and ventilator used. These can be minimized by careful attention to mask fit, pressure titration, strap tension, patient comfort, and effective communication with the patient. Nonetheless, with present technology, some failures are inevitable. Air leaks, mainly through the mouth, occur very commonly during use of nasal NPPV, may occasionally interfere with ability to assist ventilation, and ap- pears to impair sleep quality. Rebreathing is associated with bilevel- type ventilator use, and may also interfere with ability to ventilate effectively, but it has not been studied sufficiently in non-laboratory settings to fully understand its clinical significance. Major complica- tions of NPPV, including aspiration pneumonia, hypotension, baro- trauma, and respiratory arrest are, fortunately, quite unusual. Exclu- sion of inappropriate candidates and careful attention to patients during initiation help to minimize complications and assure the optimal use of NPPV. Also, technological improvements in interfaces and venti- lators are likely to lower intolerance rates in the future. However, nothing replaces the participation of dedicated, skilled, knowledgeable, and patient caregivers in optimizing the success rate of NPPV.

References

1. American Respiratory Care Foundation. Consensus Conference: non-invasive positive pressure ventilation. Resp Care 1997;42:364-369.
2. Brochard L, Mancebo J, Wysocki M, et al. Noninvasive ventilation for acute exacerbations of chronic obstructive pulmonary disease. N Engl J Med 1995;333:817-822.
3. Celikel T, Sungur M, Ceyhan B, Karakurt S. Comparison of noninvasive positive pressure ventilation with standard medical therapy in hypercapnic acute respiratory failure. Chest 1998;114:1636-1642.
4. Hill NS. Complications of noninvasive positive pressure ventilation. Respir Care 1997;42:432-442.
5. Ellis ER, McCauley VB, Mellis C, Sullivan CE. Treatment of alveolar hypoventilation in a six-year-old girl with intermittent positive pressure ventilation through a nose mask. Am Rev Respir Dis 1987;136:188-191.
6. Bach JR, Alba A, Mosher R, et al. Intermittent positive pressure ventilation via nasal access in the management of respiratory insufficiency. Chest 1987;92:168-170.
7. Navalesi P, Fanfulla F, Frigerio P, et al. Physiologic evaluation of noninvasive mechanical ventilation delivered by three types of masks in patients with chronic hypercapnic respiratory failure. Crit Care Med 2000; 28:1785-1790.
8. Meduri GU, Abou-Shala N, Fox RC, et al. Noninvasive face mask mechanical ventilation in patients with acute hypercapnic respiratory failure. Chest 1991;100:445-454.
9. Bach JR, Alba AS, Saporito LR. Intermittent positive pressure ventilation via the mouth as an alternative to tracheostomy for 257 ventilator users. Chest 1993;103:174-182.
10. Leger P, Jennequin J, Gerard M, et al. Home positive pressure ventilation via nasal mask for patients with neuromuscular weakness or restrictive lung or chest wall deformities. Respir Care 1989;34:73-77.
11. Hendrix TR. The motility of the alimentary canal. In Mountcastle VB (ed). Medical Physiology. 14th ed. St. Louis, Mosby, 1980, pp 1330-1332.
12. Dreyfuss D, Saumon G. Ventilator-induced lung injury: lessons from experimental studies. Am J Respir Crit Care Med 1998;157:294-323.
13. Richards GN, Cistulli PA, Ungar G, et al. Mouth leak with nasal continuous positive airway pressure increases nasal airway resistance. Am J Respir Crit Care Med 1996;154 182-186.
14. Wood KE, Flaten AL, Backes WJ. Inspissated secretions: a life-threatening complication of prolonged noninvasive ventilation. Respir Care 2000; 45;491-493.
15. Bach JR. Update and perspectives on noninvasive respiratory muscle aids. Part 2: the expiratory muscle aids. Chest 1994;105:1538-1544.

16. Pollack C Jr, Torres MT, Alexander L. Feasibility study of the use of bilevel positive airway pressure for respiratory support in the emergency department. Ann Emerg Med 1996;27:189-192.
17. Antonelli M, Conti G, Rocco M, et al. A comparison of noninvasive positive-pressure ventilation and conventional mechanical ventilation in patients with acute respiratory failure. N Engl J Med 1998;339:429-435.
18. Bradley DT, Holloway RM, McLaughlin PR, et al. Cardiac output response to continuous positive airway pressure in congestive heart failure. Am Rev Resp Dis 1992;145:377-382.
19. Mehta S, Jay GD, Woolard RH, et al. Randomized prospective trial of bilevel versus continuous positive airway pressure in acute pulmonary edema. Crit Care Med 1997;25:620-628.
20. Plant PK, Owen JL, Elliott MW. Early use of noninvasive ventilation for acute exacerbations of chronic obstructive pulmonary disease on general respiratory wards: a multicenter randomized controlled trial. Lancet 2000;355:1931-1935.
21. Wood KA, Lewis L, Von Harz B, Kollef MH. The use of noninvasive positive pressure ventilation in the emergency department. Chest 1998; 113:1339-1346.
22. Ambrosino N, Foglio K, Rubini F, et al. Noninvasive mechanical ventilation in acute respiratory failure due to chronic obstructive pulmonary disease: correlates for success. Thorax 1995;50:755-757.
23. Criner GJ, Brennan K, Travaline JM, Kreimer D. Efficacy and compliance with noninvasive positive pressure ventilation in patients with chronic respiratory failure. Chest 1999;116:667-675.
24. Bonmarchand G, Chevron V, Chopin C, et al. Increased initial flow rate reduces inspiratory work of breathing during pressure support ventilation in patients with exacerbation of chronic obstructive pulmonary disease. Intensive Care Med 1996;22:1147-1154.
25. Jubran A, Van de Graffe WB, Tobin MJ. Variability of patient-ventilator interaction with pressure support ventilation in patients with chronic obstructive pulmonary disease. Am J Respir Crit Care Med 1995;152:129-136.
26. Calderini E, Confalonieri M, Puccio PG, et al. Patient-ventilator asynchrony during noninvasive ventilation: the role of expiratory trigger. Intensive Care Med 1999;25:662-667.
27. Hill NS. Clinical applications of body ventilators. Chest 1986;90:897-905.
28. Jounieaux V, Aubert G, Dury M, et al. Effects of nasal positive-pressure hyperventilation on the glottis in normal awake subjects. J Appl Physiol 1995;79:176-185.
29. Jounieaux V, Aubert G, Dury M, et al. Effects of nasal positive-pressure hyperventilation on the glottis in normal sleeping subjects. J Appl Physiol 1995;79:186-183.
30. Bach JR, Dominique R, Leger P, et al: Sleep fragmentation in kyphoscoliotic individuals with alveolar hypoventilation treated by NPPV. Chest 1995;107:1552-1558.
31. Meyer TJ, Pressman MR, Benditt J, et al. Air leaking through the mouth during nocturnal nasal ventilation: effect on sleep quality. Sleep 1997; 20:561-569.

32. Ferguson GT, Gilmartin M. CO_2 rebreathing during BiPAP ventilatory assistance. Am J Respir Crit Care Med 1995;151:1126-1135.
33. Lofaso F, Brochard L, Touchard D, et al. Evaluation of carbon dioxide rebreathing during pressure support ventilation with BiPAP devices. Chest 1995;108:772-778.
34. Hill NS, Carlisle CC, Kramer NR. Does the exhalation valve really matter during bilevel nasal ventilation? Am J Respir Crit Care Med 1997; 155:A408.

Chapter 11

Program Development, Costs, Resource Utilization, and Outcomes Assessment for Noninvasive Ventilation

DeLynn Johnston, B.S., R.R.T.,
Nicholas S. Hill, M.D.

Introduction

Noninvasive ventilation has been one of the most rapidly expanding applications for mechanical ventilation over the past decade. In acute care hospitals, up to 23% of patients treated with mechanical ventilation in medical intensive care units (ICUs) receive noninvasive positive pressure ventilation (NPPV) during part of their hospitalization.[1] In the long-term care setting, a recent Minnesota survey revealed that 47% of the increase in the number of home ventilator users between 1992 and 1997 was attributable to NPPV.[2] This rapid increase in use has been fueled by the desire of clinicians to provide the optimal form of ventilator support to their patients in terms of comfort, safety, and convenience, while maximizing the efficiency of utilization. In order to achieve these aims, it is necessary for clinicians to organize both inpatient and outpatient NPPV programs, with policies for proper application and maintenance of equipment, as well as patient monitoring schedules to detect and deal with adverse side effects and complications. Programs cannot be run unless they are financially viable, so costs and reimbursement policies must be tracked, and outcomes should be assessed to determine whether objectives are being met.

NPPV Program Development

Acute Care Setting

An NPPV program in the acute setting should begin with staff education. Physicians should familiarize themselves with patient selec-

From *Noninvasive Positive Pressure Ventilation: Principles and Applications,* edited by Nicholas S. Hill. © 2001, Futura Publishing Company, Inc., Armonk, NY.

tion criteria, nurses should gain experience in caring for patients receiving NPPV, and therapists must be fully knowledgeable in the various kinds of equipment and their applications. Attendance at courses and workshop sessions is helpful, and manufacturers will provide in-service training to practitioners on the recommended uses of their products. However, nothing replaces the experience gained with application to patients. Clinicians at centers with minimal use of NPPV are encouraged to seek experience at other centers where NPPV is more routine, and then apply this experience at their own centers. Equipment to be used for NPPV should be stored, in a user-ready condition, near the emergency department or ICU. In addition, a bag containing a variety of interface sizes of types should be suspended from the NPPV ventilator.

In addition to gaining experience, staff members who administer NPPV should develop policies regarding patient selection, NPPV application, and monitoring. Although these policies should be tailored to the needs of the individual institution, one such policy used at the authors' institution for application of NPPV is exemplified in the Appendix. A program should be in place to educate patients who are to be sent home from the hospital with NPPV to show them how to apply the equipment. A dedicated team for initiation of NPPV is ideal, and implementation is best situated in a respiratory step-down unit if available. The hospital team should contact a home respiratory care vendor and establish a liaison prior to patient discharge. The vendor should bring home equipment to the hospital and ensure that the home respiratory therapist becomes familiar with the patient before discharge. Suggestions for follow-up are listed in Table 1. In areas where home respiratory vendors are unavailable, alternative means of home follow-up should be established, such as home visits by a hospital-based nurse or therapist.

Long-Term Applications

The type of program developed to maintain NPPV for long-term applications depends on the location and resources available in the particular community or country. Long-term care facilities should develop expertise in the management of patients on NPPV. Most such facilities have respiratory therapists and nurses on staff who may require additional training and experience to become skilled at the application of NPPV, but this is not difficult if these individuals are already experienced in long-term invasive ventilation. In many ways, administration of NPPV is simpler than that of invasive ventilation

Table 1
Guidelines for Follow-up of
Patients Receiving Long-Term Noninvasive Ventilation

1. Weekly home visits by respiratory therapist for first 3 weeks, then monthly, to check/review:
   Ventilator pressures
   Condition of ventilator/mask
   Ventilator timer for compliance
   Function of ventilator and mask placement with patient and family
   Equipment care and maintenance
   Emergency plan
2. Monthly follow-up by physician for 3–4 months, then at least twice yearly, to check:
   Symptoms
   Vital signs
   Hours of use
   Problems with tolerance, ventilator, mask
   Gas exchange: oximetry or end-tidal CO_2; arterial blood gases once usage > 4 hr/24 hr
   Nocturnal oximetry after 1–2 months if patient sleeping > 4h/24h using device
   Recommendations for changes in pressures or equipment; communicate with home respiratory therapist

because there is no requirement for tracheostomy tube maintenance or suctioning. On the other hand, many patients using long-term NPPV, particularly those with neuromuscular disease, have special needs for positioning and placement of the interface and for removal and resumption of ventilation, so demands on nursing staff may still be formidable.

For patients in the United States who use NPPV at home, ventilator care is usually directed by a pulmonary specialist or, on occasion, a physiatrist.[3] Patients contact the physician by phone when there are problems and also make occasional office visits. Most of the follow-up at home is carried out by visiting nurses and respiratory therapists employed by home respiratory care vendors. These professionals also communicate with the physician when problems, or the need for changes, arise. In countries where they are available, home respiratory therapists skilled in the administration of NPPV are critically important for successful adaptation of the patient; frequent home visits are conducted initially to ensure adequate compliance and to anticipate and prevent problems. The home-based program should formulate policies regarding the type and frequency of patient follow-up and ventilator maintenance. Examples of guidelines for follow-up are shown in Table 1. Some countries (i.e., France) have centralized ventilator programs that have standardized the type of care delivered and have central monitoring mechanisms that keep track of morbidity and mortality rates.[4]

Costs and Reimbursement

Acute Setting

Investigators have assessed costs in a number of different ways. Kramer et al.[5] of the United States examined hospital charges in their randomized, controlled study of nasal BiPAP ventilation in patients with various forms of acute respiratory failure. Total charges averaged $37,000 in the NPPV group and $40,000 in the control group, with no significant differences among all patients or within the subgroup of patients with chronic obstructive pulmonary disease (COPD). The lack of differences is not surprising, considering that average hospital length of stay, the single most important determinant of hospital charges in the United States, was similar in NPPV–treated patients and controls.

Nava et al.[6] of Italy examined costs of NPPV as determined by an accounting of time expenditure by medical personnel, and charges were divided into direct and indirect cost components (Table 2). Direct costs were considered laboratory tests and salaries for personnel, and indirect costs included overhead for laundry, heating, medical equipment costs, and so on. Based on these calculations, NPPV was estimated

Table 2
Total Daily Costs of Acute Application of NPPV*

Noninvasive		$806
Invasive		$864

	Percent of Costs	
Category	Noninvasive	Invasive
Personnel	36	36
X-rays	8.5	6.5
Pharmacy	8.5	9
Supplies	8	10
Laboratory	7	9
Indirect Costs	21	21
Others	11	8.5

*Total costs of the first 48 hours of NIMV and InMV expressed as daily costs (upper part) and breakdown by category (lower part).
Adapted from reference 5.

to cost $806 per day while invasive ventilation was $865 per day, a statistically nonsignificant difference. In addition, there were no significant differences with regard to the percent of costs attributable to personnel costs, laboratory or x-ray expenses, or other costs.

Although one would expect a therapy that has the potential of shortening hospital length of stay to lower costs as well, this has been difficult to demonstrate convincingly. Part of the problem is that studies that have shown shortened lengths of hospital stay have not examined costs.[7,8] Also, the methods that have examined costs have generally relied on hospital charges rather than actual costs, and this methodology is notoriously inaccurate.

Regardless of whether or not costs of NPPV are lower than those of invasive ventilation, the question of reimbursement is perhaps more germane to the current health care climate in the United States. Even if a therapy is less costly than the alternative, it may not be preferable economically if it is reimbursed at much lower rates. In a 1995 study, Criner et al.[9] showed that patients treated with NPPV in their respiratory care unit were classified using diagnosis-related group codes that undervalued the expenses of their care. They found that 82% of patients treated with NPPV incurred financial losses for the institution, averaging $9,701 per patient. These authors recommended the creation of a new code that would adequately reimburse for the expense of caring for a patient with NPPV, but this has not yet been done. In the meantime, until this change occurs, NPPV will remain a modality that can improve patient outcomes and may be cheaper for the institution overall, but idiosyncrasies of the American reimbursement system may penalize some institutions for using it. The issue of reimbursement has not received much attention outside of the United States, but undoubtedly varies between countries.

Chronic Setting

Beyond the acute care setting, the ideal setting for patients using NPPV is in the home.[3] Compared with invasive mechanical ventilation via a tracheostomy, NPPV greatly facilitates care, eliminating the need for frequent suctioning or care of the airway. On the other hand, depending on the availability of family members or significant others to help, and the needs of the individual for assistance with activities of daily living, costs of home care can vary tremendously. In one of the few studies to analyze these costs, Bach et al.[10] found that on average, costs of patients receiving NPPV at home are much less than those of patients receiving invasive ventilation in a chronic care facility. Costs of in-patient care for 30 ventilator-assisted individuals (VAIs) averaged $718.80 per patient per day, based on Medicare reimbursement rates. When the patients were discharged home on noninvasive ventilation, average cost declined 77% to $235.13 per patient per day. This cost estimate was comprised mainly of personnel expenses, amounting to 81% of the total. Ventilator equipment rental expenses were the next greatest category, and other costs for supplies and disposables were inconsequential.

Although these results support the contention that NPPV reduces the costs of care, it should be borne in mind that the subjects of Bach's study were special in that their caregivers were trained but had no credentials to provide ventilator care. Such attendants have not been legitimized in many states, where only attendants with credentials are allowed to care for VAIs. The requirement for credentialed attendants may double personnel costs. If patients using NPPV require more than 12 hours per 24 hours of skilled nursing care, costs can easily exceed $500 per day. Nonetheless, costs for long-term NPPV are almost certainly less than those for similarly impaired individuals using invasive ventilation because of the elimination of the need for tracheostomy care or suctioning and the reduced likelihood of pneumonia.

Health Care Financing Agency Guidelines

Recently, the medical directors of the Durable Medical Equipment Regional Carriers (DMERC), the group under the Health Care Financing Agency (HCFA) that is directly responsible for setting reimbursement policy for Medicare, have revised clinical indicators for the reimbursement of NPPV for long-term care. Although Medicare covers a minority of health care consumers in the United States, it is the single largest insurer, and its policies influence those of other payers. The desire for revision of the reimbursement policy was driven by rapidly increasing billings for NPPV from home care companies and HCFA's concern that some of these applications were inappropriate. A consensus group of international experts was convened by the National Association of Medical Directors of Respiratory Care (NAMDRC) in February 1998, and the Consensus Report was recently published in *Chest*.[11] Based largely on the consensus group's recommendations, the medical directors of the DMERC produced a draft of proposed clinical indicators for NPPV.[12]

In the draft proposal, reimbursement for NPPV was divided into 2 equipment categories: KO 532 for respiratory assist devices (RADs) lacking a backup rate (i.e., spontaneous or S mode) and KO 533 for devices with a backup rate (i.e., the assist/control or the spontaneous/ timed mode). The former devices are considered to require less maintenance and are reimbursed as a capped rental, with a lower reimbursement monthly for a total of 15 months. The devices with a backup rate are considered to require frequent maintenance and monitoring, and are reimbursed at a substantially higher rate indefinitely.

The DMERC identified 3 clinical categories for reimbursement: restrictive thoracic disorders, COPD, and nocturnal hypoventilation (or sleep apnea). Patients with restrictive thoracic disorders qualified for either KO 532 or 533 devices at the discretion of the clinician if they had symptoms of chronic hypoventilation despite maximal medical therapy, and had either daytime gas exchange abnormalities, evidence of nocturnal hypoventilation, or severe pulmonary dysfunction (Table 3). It should be emphasized that the nocturnal oximetry study for these patients does not require use of supplemental O_2. In fact, O_2 supplementation without ventilatory assistance in these patients can lead to dangerous elevations of CO_2 and should be used only with caution.[13]

For patients with COPD, the DMERC guidelines require substantial daytime CO_2 retention (Table 4). The specific threshold for $PaCO_2$ has been a matter of some debate. The NAMDRC consensus group suggested a $PaCO_2$ of at least 50 mm Hg as a reasonable threshold value in view of the variability between studies.[11] Initially, the DMERC guidelines adopted a $PaCO_2$ of at least 55 mm Hg as the threshold value. However, this has since been reduced to 52 mm Hg when it was pointed out that the higher value would have excluded one third of the patients who benefited from NPPV in the one controlled trial with favorable results.[14]

Table 3

Health Care Financing Agency Guidelines for Use of NPPV in Restrictive Thoracic Disease

---

A. Documentation of ventilatory restriction due to neuromuscular disease or chest wall deformity, *and*
B. 1. Daytime $PaCO_2 \geq 45mm$ Hg, *or*
   2. Sleep oximetry showing O_2 sat < 88% for > 5 consecutive minutes at usual FiO_2, *and*
C. COPD does not contribute significantly.

Table 4
Health Care Financing Agency
Guidelines for Use of NPPV in Severe COPD

A. Daytime $PaCO_2 \geq 52$ mm Hg while patient breathes usual FiO_2, *and*
B. Sleep oximetry shows O_2 sat, $< 88\%$ for > 5 consecutive minutes at usual FiO_2, *and*
C. Obstructive sleep apnea has been considered and excluded.

The DMERC guidelines also require that obstructive sleep apnea be considered and excluded, and that nocturnal oximetry be performed with the patient using the usual FiO_2. In order to qualify, patients must have an O_2 desaturation $< 88\%$ for at least 5 consecutive minutes as a means of demonstrating nocturnal hypoventilation. Patients who meet these guidelines will be reimbursed for NPPV, but only at the lower KO 532 capped rental rate for a 3-month requisite trial. At the end of 2 months, patients will be continued on NPPV if their physicians certify that they have clinically improved and are using the device for at least 20 hours weekly. If patients are not clinically improved, switching to a ventilator with a backup rate can be done if a sleep study demonstrates improvement in gas exchange during use of the assist/control mode.

The effectiveness of NPPV in severe stable COPD has been debated,[15] and the HCFA guidelines are considered excessively severe by some clinicians. First, there are no data to support the guideline requiring sustained O_2 desaturation as an indicator of nocturnal hypoventilation. The Meecham Jones et al. study[14] showed that the improvement in nocturnal hypoventilation after initiation of NPPV correlated with the improvement in daytime $PaCO_2$, suggesting that nocturnal hypoventilation might help to identify COPD patients who are likely to respond favorably to NPPV. However, it did not demonstrate that this hypoventilation correlated with any parallel changes in O_2 saturation, nor has the sensitivity or specificity of a 5-minute desaturation episode in detecting nocturnal hypoventilation ever been tested. Thus, it is possible that patients who otherwise might benefit will be denied coverage because they fail to desaturate enough. The NAMDRC consensus group had suggested similar guidelines with regard to O_2 desaturation, but only for patients with $PaCO_2$s between 50 mm Hg and 54 mm Hg. Further, the recommendation by the consensus group that patients with multiple hospitalizations for hypercapnic respiratory failure be given a trial of NPPV was not incorporated into the HCFA guidelines.

Finally, and perhaps of most concern, the 2-month requisite trial at the lower reimbursement rate will likely compromise the economic feasibility of NPPV delivery to COPD patients (who initially require frequent visits from home respiratory therapists for ventilator and mask adjustments[9]). The net effect of these guidelines will be to restrict the use of NPPV for COPD patients.

The clinical indicators for NPPV in patients with sleep apnea, in contrast to those for COPD patients, have generated relatively little controversy (Table 5). These call for use of a "bilevel" type device without a backup rate as long as the patient has obstructive sleep apnea documented on a polysomnogram and evidence of nocturnal hypoventilation as suggested by sustained O_2 desaturations (>5 min) despite continuous positive airway pressure (CPAP) therapy. If central sleep apnea is demonstrated, then a backup rate can be added.

These reimbursement policies will determine, to a large extent, the use of NPPV for long-term application in the United States, for the foreseeable future. Modifications in the policies are likely as new information becomes available. However, until studies are completed that convincingly demonstrate efficacy of NPPV for patients with COPD, the policies will likely continue to limit use for this patient population.

Monitoring Outcomes for NPPV

What Are Outcomes?

Outcomes are the result of an intervention or specific process. A favorable outcome achieves a defined goal. From a clinical viewpoint, outcomes are the measurable changes in an individual or defined popu-

---

Table 5
Health Care Financing Agency
Guidelines for Use of NPPV in Central Sleep Apnea

A. Central sleep apnea demonstrated on a facility-based polysomnogram, *and*
B. Obstructive sleep apnea (OSA) excluded as a major contributor of hypoventilation, *or*
C. If OSA is a major contributor, CPAP has been tried and failed, *and*
D. O_2 sat < 88% for 5 > consecutive minutes at 2 L/min O_2 or usual FiO_2 *and*
E. Significant improvement of sleep-associated hypoventilation is documented.

lation resulting from specific interventions. They measure the effectiveness of the intervention and/or the provider, and the impact these have on the patient. Outcome monitoring provides a larger perspective on health care delivery than is ordinarily available to the individual practitioner. By monitoring outcomes, benefits of the services provided can be evaluated.

Outcomes measurement is the process of gathering and evaluating the results of an intervention, event, or process. It involves the continuous or regular tracking of patient and health care information over time. The time periods for measuring outcomes are both short-term and long-term. Outcomes measurement offers a method to determine the operational performance and effectiveness of a health care provider and/or the care paths utilized.

Outcomes research tracks and quantifies outcomes within a specific patient population and encourages the evaluation of a variety of care practices. Health care outcomes research is a vehicle that facilitates the examination of interdisciplinary care, identifying appropriate care processes that draw practitioners closer to the discovery and use of best practices. In this regard, outcomes research is a fundamental component of quality improvement initiatives.

Outcomes management is a research-based process of measurement and analysis of health outcomes and dissemination of health outcomes information to appropriate decision makers, namely patients, providers, and payers. It facilitates discovery and implementation of the best practices through practice standardization, benchmarking, continuous quality monitoring, and improvement. The goal of outcomes management is to deliver high-quality, cost-effective care as efficiently as possible by using critical pathways. From the provider's perspective, it is an ongoing quest for best practice; from the payer's perspective, it makes for more rational allocation of resources within diagnostic groups or for high risk subgroups of patients.

Why Are Outcomes Important?

With increasing pressure on our health care system to control costs, there are great demands on health care providers to justify the expenditure of scarce resources on patient care and to demonstrate that health care practices are benefiting patients at the lowest possible cost. A number of forces are spurring this movement including:

- The shift of reimbursement to more capitated arrangements.

- The assumption of risk by providers.

- The increase in managed care coverage of products.

- The increase in integrated health care delivery systems.

- The concerns about maintaining quality of care in light of economic pressures to improve efficiency.

The Joint Commission on Accreditation of Health Care Organizations (JCAHO) has also joined this movement. The JCAHO supports implementation of best practices through benchmarking and quality improvement via their new performance measurement requirements, ORYX: The Next Evolution in Accreditation. ORYX incorporates performance measures into the accreditation process. The JCAHO describes this initiative as the critical link between accreditation and the outcomes of patient care. For the first time, the Joint Commission will survey the process by which health care organizations use data to improve patient care. The ORYX process for accredited health care organizations is being implemented in hospitals, long-term care facilities, home care, hospices, and by ambulatory care and long-term care providers.[16]

What Outcomes Are Usually Monitored?

Traditional health care outcomes are patient morbidity and mortality rates. The concept of health care-related outcomes has expanded the list to encompass additional elements such as clinical, financial, functional or health status, satisfaction, and performance indicators. These can be categorized in several different ways: organizational, patient, and disease outcomes; financial, service, and clinical outcomes; and utilization, access, and health status outcomes. The various category groupings are reflective of the viewpoint of the case manager, health care provider, or the payer/managed care organization.

Clinical outcome measures track changes in anatomic and physiologic findings, including adverse results and specific changes in a patient's physical condition (Table 6, A). Based on a clinician's assessment, these results are taken from the patient record, either through chart audit or the concurrent data collection available with point of care automation. Common clinical measures for patients with respiratory disorders include, but are not limited to, vital signs, physical findings, arterial blood gases, pulse oximetry, end-tidal CO_2 measurements,

Table 6
Outcome Data Sets Commonly Collected by Health Care Agencies

A. Physiologic and Clinical Measures	B. Financial Measures
Vital signs	Length of stay
Arterial blood gases	Number of ICU days
Pulmonary function tests	Avoidance of intubation
Nocturnal oximetry	Mechanical ventilation time
Hours of therapy use	Hospital re-admissions
Infection rate	ED admissions
Other complications	Physician visits
Shortness of breath	Resource utilization rates
Respiratory disturbance index	Complication
Need for supplemental O_2	Staff resource allocation
End-tidal CO_2	Need for caregivers at home
Morbidity	Total cost of care
Mortality	

C. Patient/Family Health Status and Satisfaction Measures	D. Service/Performance Measures
	Frequency of clinician visits
Activities of daily living	Visits
Dyspnea scores	Equipment maintenance
Exercise tolerance	Equipment failures
Emotional status	Incorrect deliveries
Perceived quality of life	Education assessment
Mental status	Documentation tracking
Anxiety level	Emergency service calls
Depression	Delay in responding to calls
Comfort levels	Patient complaints
Evaluation of care received	
Ability for self-care	

shortness of breath, respiratory disturbance index, need for supplemental oxygen, infection and complication rates, and morbidity and mortality.

Financial outcome measures include costs of care, charges, and reimbursements that may have little relation to one another (Table 6, B). Related outcomes include measures of resource utilization, such as length of hospital stay, number of ventilator days, number of days in the ICU, ICU rebound/avoidance, hospital admissions/readmissions, emergency department, physician's office, and home care visits, and staff resource allocation. Additional factors affecting cost of care include appropriateness, efficacy, utilization, and the prices of services provided.

The patient's functional or health status (Table 6, C), sometimes referred to as physical status, typically involves survey questionnaires to obtain the patient's assessment of his/her health and quality of life. These surveys offer the dual benefit of standardization and cross-continuum measurement. Health status outcomes can assess and compare the results achieved by various health services in both institutional- and community-based settings. Health status is often gauged by the ability to perform activities of daily living, the extent of self-care, exercise tolerance, a resumption of gainful employment, and overall capacity for activity and accomplishment. Examples of exercise tolerance measurement tools include the 6 Minute Walk Test (6MWT), 12 Minute Walk Test (12MWT), the Shuttle Walk Test (SWT), and treadmill or cycle endurance times.

Subjective indices such as dyspnea scores, both at rest and with varying levels of activity, can also be included in the assessment of the patient's functional status. Multiple measurement tools are available to assess and compare dyspnea levels before, during, and after intervention. They include the Borg Scale of Perceived Dyspnea, Baseline and Transition Dyspnea Indexes (BDI and TDI), American Thoracic Society Dyspnea Scale, The University of California, San Diego, Shortness of Breath Questionnaire (SOBQ), and the Visual Analog Scale (VAS).[17]

Patient satisfaction measures an important aspect of quality; it serves as an index of a provider's ability to meet or exceed the patient's expectations for services provided. However, patient satisfaction has some limitations as an indicator of overall quality. It is dependent on the patient's understanding and expectations of the service and is therefore subject to individual bias and misinterpretation. Patient satisfaction is assessed by measuring multiple components including quality of life, emotional status, mental status, anxiety level, depression, and comfort level. Often, these are combined into a composite score that gives an overall perception of the patient's quality of life.

Commonly used tools for assessing satisfaction and quality of life include customized patient satisfaction surveys and the Quality of Well-Being (QWB) Scale. To evaluate specifically for anxiety, the Speilberger State-Trait Anxiety Inventory (STAI) can be used. Tools to evaluate depression and emotional outcomes include the Geriatric Depression Score (GDS), Hospital Anxiety and Depression Scale (HAD), Mood Adjective Checklist (MACL), and the Center for Epidemiologic Studies' Depression (CESD) Scale.

Overall health status assessment tools that consider multiple facets of health status in the patient's quality of life include the SF-36 (which has multiple variants) and the Sickness Impact Profile (SIP). Several survey instruments designed specifically to assess the health status of patients with respiratory disease include the St. George's

Respiratory Questionnaire (SGRQ), the Chronic Respiratory Questionnaire (CRQ), Breathing Problems Questionnaire (BPQ), and the Seattle Obstructive Lung Disease Questionnaire (SOLQ).[18] Debate exists as to whether there is any advantage in using a respiratory-specific questionnaire as opposed to a general quality of life questionnaire. To choose the most appropriate, a variety of assessment tools should be evaluated, considering the questions being asked, the types of patients involved, the information sought, and the difficulty in administering the questionnaire relevant to the patient population and the resources of the surveyor.

Satisfaction is not only relevant to the patient and family, but also to payers and employers. Employers rely on the payer industry to manage their benefit costs and so, are interested in health care outcomes as well. These groups are now demanding reliable, valid outcome data to determine if the value of the services they are receiving justifies their expenditures. Their perception of value consists of high-quality and cost-efficient service as well as an overall level of satisfaction for their clients.

Performance Indicators

Home care providers use performance indicators to assess the quality and cost effectiveness of the products and services provided to the patient and family (Table 6, D). Measuring service performance requires an understanding of the key performance areas for the services to be evaluated. These key areas should be reviewed to determine which factors are important to the success or effectiveness of those services. These may include such indicators as the timeliness of service delivery, cost efficiencies and inefficiencies, appropriate cost-containment measures, error recognition and elimination, and the effectiveness of patient and family instruction, education, and counseling. Additional elements include equipment maintenance and failures, unscheduled service calls, and visits by clinicians to assess the patient's status in his/her own environment. Service performance has a dramatic effect on the cost of providing health care. Poorly organized or ineffectively provided health care can adversely affect clinical outcomes and unnecessarily increase overall costs.

The scope of performance indicators differs among the various settings in which care is provided. Among critical care, acute care, subacute care, and home care sites, the performance measures used are based on similar concepts, but the specific formats are unique to each environment. In order to accurately measure and compare different services provided in each environment, there must be standardized questions and indicators. The need for consistent, reliable, and valid tools is being addressed by several national organizations such as Gallup, Picker Institute, and the National Committee for Quality Assurance. Standardization of survey instruments, data collection, and analysis make benchmarking efforts feasible.

What Is the Future in Outcomes Research?

The current medical environment, with its pressure to reduce health care costs and improve the quality and delivery of health care, will ensure a central role for future outcome investigations. The challenges to practitioners are 4-fold:

- to identify the most important issues or questions requiring investigations;

- to define the most appropriate outcomes for study;

- to train and develop clinical investigators for outcomes research;

- to identify and develop funding mechanisms to support such investigations.[19]

Determining what outcomes to measure is difficult because many are qualitative in nature, change over time, and vary depending on the patient subgroup. Ideally, randomized, controlled trials should be done to assess clinical efficacy, but many situations are not amenable to such trials. Randomized trials on small populations are subject to chance variations and suffer from inadequate statistical power. Observational studies are subject to bias and confounding factors, such as variability in patient characteristics, which may affect outcomes. In addition, many chronic illnesses have unpredictable courses unrelated to treatment.[20] Research should be designed to avoid methodological problems such as a small sample size, lack of adequate control populations, incompletely validated outcome measures, and the absence of prospective data collection.[21] The goal in outcomes research should be to strive for the highest level of evidence feasible.[22]

What Outcomes Are Relevant to NPPV?

Elimination of a permanent artificial airway increases patient convenience and independence, simplifies care, and reduces costs by obviating the need for tracheostomy, suctioning supplies, and the highly skilled personnel necessary to manage these patients.[23] As with many clinical issues involving diverse patient populations, randomized, controlled studies are difficult to fund and implement. However, the large accumulating body of experience with NPPV suggests its wider application is worth further outcomes research and outcomes management. This facilitates the identification of best practices, enhances disease management, increases patient self-care levels, and addresses the needs of the changing health care environment.

The literature on NPPV reveals an ever-growing body of evidence related to the outcomes of this advance in the treatment of respiratory disorders. Favorable outcomes have been reported in clinical, financial, functional status, patient satisfaction, and quality of life areas. Most frequently noted results include improved gas exchange, improved sleep, avoidance of intubation, reduced duration of mechanical ventilation, shortened length of stay, and decreased mortality.

How Should an Outcome Measurement Program Be Implemented?

The specific measures selected to assess outcomes depend on the role the outcomes assessor plays in servicing a patient with NPPV. Acute care practitioners, home care providers, and third-party payers are all interested in outcomes from different viewpoints and, as such, need different data sets. In establishing an NPPV program, the outcomes chosen for monitoring will depend on the type of information needed. This can vary from one care setting to another and also related to the entity collecting the data. For example, an acute care practitioner's primary interest might be focused on clinical and financial indicators. Home care providers" need for data may involve financial and service or performance indicators. Third-party payers often look for financial data relating therapeutic efficacy and cost efficiency. Even patient satisfaction will take on differing tones, based on these various viewpoints. Despite these differences in data needs, however, a great deal of overlap exists across the spectrum of outcomes information.

Summary and Conclusions

With the increasing use of NPPV, programs and policies should be implemented that aim to optimize effectiveness and resource utilization. Knowledge of cost and reimbursement issues is essential to running a successful program. In addition, it is important that successful programs monitor outcomes. Outcome monitoring provides useful data for measuring clinical efficacy and financial effectiveness, and also helps to identify operational problems. The data that is collected can provide averages for benchmarking that can then be used to establish goals for operational improvements as well as identification of clinical care paths and best practices. Appropriately applied, this leads to improved health care across the continuum of involved parties. Outcome monitoring should be included as part of any program of NPPV so that clinicians can rapidly identify and promptly deal with potential problems, helping to assure that the goals of the program will be achieved.

References

1. Meduri GU, Turner RE, Abou-Shala N, et al. Noninvasive positive pressure ventilation via face mask. Chest 1996;109:179-193.
2. Adams AB, Shapiro R, Marini JJ. Changing prevalence of chronically ventilator-assisted individuals in Minnesota: increases, characteristics, and the use of noninvasive ventilation. Respir Care 1998;43:643-649.
3. Make BJ, Hill NS, Goldberg AI, et al. Mechanical ventilation beyond the intensive care. Chest 1998;113:289S-344S.
4. Antadir CE. Association nationale pous le traitment a domicile de l'insuffisance respiratoire chronique. Observatory. Data of January 1, 1996. Trends. Paris, Antadir, 1997.
5. Kramer N, Meyer TJ, Meharg J, et al. Randomized, prospective trial of noninvasive positive pressure ventilation in acute respiratory failure. Am J Respir Crit Care Med 1995;151:1799-1806.
6. Nava S, Evangesliti I, Rampulla C, et al. Human and financial costs of noninvasive mechanical ventilation in patients affected by COPD and acute respiratory failure. Chest 1997;111:1631-1638.
7. Brochard L, Mancebo J, Wysocki M, et al. Noninvasive ventilation for acute exacerbations of chronic obstructive pulmonary disease. N Engl J Med 1995;333:817-822.
8. Celikel T, Sungur M, Ceyhan B, Karakurt S. Comparison of noninvasive positive pressure ventilation with standard medical therapy in hypercapnic acute respiratory failure. Chest 1998;114:1636-1642.
9. Criner GJ, Kreimer DT, Tomaselli M, et al. Financial implications of noninvasive positive pressure ventilation (NPPV). Chest 1995;108:475-481.

10. Bach JR, Intintola P, Alba AS, Holland I. The ventilator-assisted individual cost analysis of institutionalization versus rehabilitation and in-home management. Chest 1992;101:26-30.
11. Consensus Conference. Clinical indications for noninvasive positive pressure ventilation in chronic respiratory failure due to restrictive lung disease, COPD, and nocturnal hypoventilation: a Consensus Conference report. Chest 1999;116:521-534.
12. Region B DMERC Supplier Manual Medical Policy. Respiratory Assist Device (RAD), Rev 20-December, 1999, pp 199-210.
13. Gay PC, Edmonds LC. Severe hypercapnia after low-flow oxygen therapy in patients with neuromuscular disease and diaphragmatic dysfunction. Mayo Clin Proc 1995;70(4):327-330.
14. Meecham Jones DJ, Paul EA, Jones PW. Nasal pressure support ventilation plus oxygen compared with oxygen therapy along in hypercapnic COPD. Am J Respir Crit Care Med 1995;152:538-544.
15. Rossi A, Hill NS. Noninvasive ventilation has been shown to be effective/ineffective in stable COPD: pro-con debate. Am J Respir Crit Care Med 2000;161:688-691.
16. Popovich ML. ORYX: the next evolution in accreditation. JCAHO Homecare Bull 1997;1:1.
17. Sassi-Dambron DE, Eakin EG, Ries AS, Kaplan RM. Treatment of dyspnea in COPD: a controlled clinical trial of dyspnea management strategies. Chest 1995;107:724-729.
18. Tu SP, McDonell MB, Spertus JA, et al. A new self-administered questionnaire to monitor health-related quality of life in patients with COPD. Chest 1997;112:614-622.
19. Kollef MH. Outcomes research in the ICU setting: is it worthwhile? Chest 1997;112:870-873.
20. Orchard C. Comparing healthcare outcomes. Br Med J 1994;308:1493-1496.
21. Zhang YC, Zhong NS. COPD and noninvasive ventilation. RT International 1995;Fall:99-104.
22. Cook DJ, et al. American College of Chest Physicians project on evidence-based medicine. Chest 1992;102:305S-311S.
23. Hill NS. Noninvasive ventilation. Pulm Perspect 1997;14:1-4.

Policy for the Implementation of NPPV for Acute Respiratory Failure

Goal

The goal is to provide noninvasive ventilation to appropriate patients with acute respiratory failure in a safe cost-effective manner, so as to avoid endotracheal intubation and reduce the attendant morbidity and mortality.

Patients

Eligible patients will have acute respiratory failure with a reasonable expectation of reversal within a few days. Typical diagnoses include, but are not limited to: COPD, CHF/acute pulmonary edema, pneumonia, asthma, postoperative respiratory failure, and do-not-intubate patients (should have reversible cause for respiratory failure).

Eligible patients are in need of ventilatory assistance as determined by:

1. Acute respiratory distress of at least moderate severity, and

2. Evidence of increased work of breathing. Tachypnea, RR > 24 breaths/min for COPD or asthma patients, RR > 30 breaths/min for pulmonary edema, pneumonia, etc.
   Accessory muscle use, or abdominal paradox and

3. Gas exchange abnormality: $PaCO_2 > 45$ mm Hg with pH < 7.35 or $PaO_2/FiO_2 \leq 200$.

Patients with any of the following are *ineligible*:

1. Respiratory arrest or immediate need for intubation

2. Medically unstable (hypotensive shock, acute myocardial infarction, uncontrolled ischemia or arrhythmias, uncontrolled upper GI bleeding, etc.)

233

3. Unable to protect airway: severe swallowing disorder and/or impaired cough, excessive secretions

4. Excessive agitation or uncooperativeness

5. Recent upper airway or esophageal surgery

6. Unable to fit mask

Equipment

"Bilevel" or "critical care" ventilator
Full face or nasal mask—variety of sizes
Headgear for mask
Artificial skin for nose
Fitting gauge for mask
Ventilator tubing
Oxygen source
Optional: humidifier

Location

Intensive Care Unit
Respiratory Care Unit
Emergency Department

Procedure
1. Explain process to patient who is sitting at 45–90° in bed.
2. Size mask using fitting gauge.
   Use forehead spacer (if applicable).
   Apply artificial skin to nose.
3. Select a ventilator.
4. Hold mask in place (while patient holds it, if possible) and connect to ventilator.
5. Initiate ventilation with pressure support mode, pressures 8–10/4–5 cm H_2O (inspiratory/expiratory).
6. Gradually increase inspiratory pressure to 10–16 cm H_2O range as tolerated; try to reduce respiratory rate.

7. Titrate O_2 via mask or T-connector (or increase FiO_2 if O_2 blender) to maintain O_2 saturation ≥ 90–92%.
8. Secure mask with headgear, avoid excessive tightening.
9. Check for air leaks, readjust mask.
10. Set backup rate at 12–16; use humidifier as needed.
11. Frequent checks for encouragement and coaching

Monitoring

Vital signs
Continuous oximetry
Sternocleidomastoid muscle activity
Patient-ventilator synchrony
Tidal/minute volume (if possible)
Occasional blood gases

Weaning Criteria

Stable vital signs
RR < 24–28 breaths/min (depending on initial RR)
FiO_2 ≤ 50% and EPAP ≤ 5 cm H_2O
O_2 saturation > 90% with $PaCO_2$ at usual level, pH > 7.35
Rapid—discontinue NPPV, monitor closely, remains off if comfortable, resume if meets initiation criteria.
Slow—gradual reduction of inspiratory pressure by 2–3 cm H_2O every 2 hours as tolerated. Watch for increased respiratory rate or sternocleidomastoid muscle activity.

Respiratory Treatments

May be given via nebulizer or metered dose inhaler with spacer during brief interruption, or may be administered "in-line" via ventilator during NPPV use.

Ventilator Malfunction

If ventilator malfunction is suspected, disconnect and initiate bag ventilation until problem is solved.

Oronasal Masks

Do not require routine nasogastric tubes.
Should have "anti-asphyxia" valves and quick release straps.

Index